DEMETRIUS ELLIS

Reflections of "Nephron Man"

A Road Map for Revitalizing the Medical Profession

5/1/2019

To Dr. Eric Goluboff

My cousin, Joel Drape, how much
affection for you personally, and much
respect for your exceptional professional
skills and expertise. I have worked in
very close collaboration with my pediatric
urology colleagues over the past 45 years and
attribute much of my own professional enrichment
to them. They also benefited countless
mutual patients with congenital and acquired
urologic disorders that were very challenging
and very vexing to their parents. and service
I thank you for your dedication
to Joe and on behalf of all your
patients. Hopefully you will enjoy reading
my book! in your
Much health, joy + fulfillment life
personal + professional

Demetrius Ellis

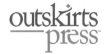

Book Dedication

My legacy to my children and grandchildren consists of several important components, one of which is this book. In addition, I dedicate this book to my wife, Irene, who supported me along every step of my career and for enriching all aspects of my life. Most of all, the book celebrates the phenomenal resiliency and courage of children everywhere who struggle to overcome serious illnesses or other life adversities and pursue a lifestyle that maximizes their chances of success in life. I commend them and endorse their efforts!

All royalties from this book are for the benefit of disadvantaged and refugee children at my birthplace, the Greek isle of Lesvos.

TABLE OF CONTENTS

Introduction

THROUGHOUT HUMAN HISTORY, no profession has been held to higher ethical and professional standards than the practice of medicine. This profession is centered on a desire to heal others, and mutual respect and trust that typically—hopefully—develop over time between patient and physician. Patients are often more willing to share their innermost secrets and maladies with physicians than with their friends, members of their families, or confessions with their priests. Developing such a strong and enduring relationship has long been regarded an essential feature of traditional medicine because of its important role in facilitating both the prevention and management of medical disorders. Thus, in the past, our society placed a high premium on doctors and on the medical profession. And, yes, physicians were well compensated for their prolonged medical education and training as well as dedication and long work hours. Hence, top college graduates often aspired to pursue a medical career.

The past half-century bears witness to transformative advances in science and technology that have resulted in longer life span and higher quality of life in nearly all Americans. By necessity, the exponential increase in scientific information together with more complex—and costly—medical care has altered the traditional model of care in a dramatic way. It has given rise to over 120 medical specialties, thus diminishing the role of primary care physicians in the evaluation and management of patients with serious disorders. Such patients are typically referred to specialists with expertise in the particular organ affected. Pediatric kidney specialists (nephrologists) such as me nearly always evaluate and treat children in large university-affiliated children's hospitals. In addition, most specialists are mandated to provide medical teaching and to advance knowledge in their respective specialty through research. These responsibilities are collectively designated as "academic medicine." In my capacity as the chief of the Division of Pediatric Nephrology, I was expected to carry out many administrative duties as well. However, throughout my forty-two-year career, I nearly always cared for patients on a daily basis—referred throughout the book as *clinical* duty. In the course of reading this book, I am certain that that you will become fully convinced that I was overworked and undercompensated. However, this was more than counterbalanced by the many enriching, interesting, and unique experiences. I truly enjoyed nearly all aspects of my career but unequivocally, contributing to the health of children and comforting their families have been my greatest rewards.

A significant portion of this book describes the circumstances that brought me together with my patients and their families, the strong bonds that were forged between us and the many emotions or feelings that we shared that transcended any socioeconomic differences. Because much of the book reflects how my interaction with patients influenced my personal development and philosophy on the practice of medicine, it represents an autobiography limited to my career that emerges indirectly largely through the narration of actual patient anecdotes and stories. Indeed, I value the words of my patients and their families above my own because, on final analysis, they are my most important teachers and discriminating critics. Both health care providers and recipients will readily identify with the trials and tribulations of the individuals in these stories. More importantly, the unique experiences and enduring relationships I had with my patients, enabled me to formulate and share with you a set of life lessons or tenets that I

Reflections of "Nephron Man"

found invaluable in my own practice of medicine (see p. 209, *Advice to residents and fellows: Strive to be the best!*).

When referring to my patients and certain medical personnel, I use names or abbreviations that obscure their real identities. My recollection of dates and events was aided by a large trough of saved letters and pictures sent to me by my patients, dating back to the start of my career, as well as formal and informal documents, newspaper articles, and other information. For purposes of giving context to the stories, I provide a brief, simplified version of the child's medical disorder. I hasten to add, however, that an emphasis on kidney disorders is unavoidable given my specialty and my admitted bias and unbridled love for the kidney. I choose to think that most physicians are equally passionate about their chosen specialty. My intention, however, is not to focus on the kidney and its disorders; these only sub-serve as a background of the stories in the book. Hence, readers who feel encumbered by medical jargon may elect to skim over these sections without detracting from the larger theme contained within each anecdote.

Similarly, the anecdotes related to the book sections on *Teaching, Research, Administration, Politics and medicine*, etc, impart a more complete perspective of my overall academic experience. I believe that most readers will find these interesting, perhaps amusing, and informative. These sections together with *My crisis in academic medicine*, may disclose less known facets of academic medicine that may be especially intriguing to younger physicians contemplating to pursue such career. Admittedly, however, non-health care providers may be less interested in learning about several of these more esoteric duties and challenges of physicians employed at university-affiliated facilities and may choose to skim through these sections.

Sadly, over the past five decades the traditional practice of medicine that I enjoyed throughout my career has been on a perilous course. It is quite apparent that many physicians from nearly all specialties have become increasingly dissatisfied and disillusioned with various aspects of their profession. At the core of this discontent are encompassing health care delivery regulations imposed on physicians by governmental and private agencies without adequate input on their part. These regulations often clash with physician values and ideals and undermine their autonomy or control over the brand of medicine they wish to deliver (see, *The changing face of the medical profession*, p. 222). Even though patients have been the beneficiaries of medical innovations, paradoxically, many of them are also dissatisfied with many aspects of their care. Hence, understanding the fundamental reasons and finding solutions to these problems is essential in insuring a healthy and effective medical profession going forward. I contend that the anecdotes and paradigms I relate herein serve to inspire physicians to refocus on getting to know the individual and not just his/her disease. This attitude together with adopting the set of tenets or principles I describe, can serve as a road map that empowers healthcare professionals to become more efficacious healers and, in the process, rediscover the joy and fulfillment that is at the core of this noble profession. The book may also be of interest to those at the crossroads of deciding to enter a medical career and to all recipients of medical care who stand to benefit from a revitalized and reinvigorated medical profession.

Because I choose to judge my success as a physician by how I am perceived by my students, patients and their families, I end the book by reflecting on my retirement and include a sampling of their letters.

Why I pursued an academic Pediatric career?

Growing up in Brooklyn, New York, I had the great fortune of having two excellent role models: my uncle Michael and his wonderful wife, Stavroula, or Voula for short. Both had a genuine affection for children, loved their work and were exemplary pediatricians. In addition, they possessed great energy, a spirit of generosity, and a good sense of humor. Thusly, they earned the respect of the families and children under their care, and in the process, they achieved wide acclaim and some measure of wealth. Along with the community at large, I admired and respected them. This motivated me to focus on my studies in the hopes of one day following in their footsteps and become a pediatrician. Thus, I always considered pediatrics, but a specialty beyond that never entered my mind until early in my medical school education.

1969 AND MEDICAL
SCHOOL AT BUFFALO

THE YEAR **1969** was the year I matriculated in medical school at the State University of New York (SUNY) at Buffalo, or UB for short, marking the start of my medical career. Because this singular milestone set me on my career path and ultimately led to the writing of this book, I wish to digress and provide a brief personal introduction and a description of the circumstances that set the stage for me to matriculate at UB.

You may be curious to learn why I elected to introduce myself to you at this early junction of the book. This is because I am keenly aware that my name and accent invariably arouse curiosity about my ethnic origin whenever I make new acquaintances like you, or on nearly all initial contacts I had with patients during my career. When I was a younger physician, I felt somewhat defensive and less compelled to explain these distinguishing features because I did not perceive either of those things to define who I was and because I considered myself an American first. As I grew older, I was less bothered by it. So, let us dispense of this. Yes, I am of Greek heritage and very proud of it. I was born on the island of Lesvos, also known as Lesbos or Mytilene, and came to the U.S. just before my thirteenth birthday. Yes, I am a *Lesbian* in the true sense of the word (which has a very different connotation in

Greek than in English). My surname was *Theodorellis*. The "*Theodor*" portion means "*God's gift*" while the "*ellis*" suffix is common to surnames of inhabitants of Lesvos. Five years after my arrival to the U.S., I took a brief American history test and an oath and was pronounced a naturalized American citizen. At that instant, I had the option of legally changing my name. This was very appealing to me, not because I wished to change my identity, but because I tended to become annoyed from having to spell my polysyllabic surname at nearly all new interactions. Thus, without informing my family, I amputated the "*Theodor*" portion and henceforth was known as "*Ellis*". Albeit unforeseen, that fortuitous act markedly facilitated the signing of perhaps millions of prescriptions and documents much later, when I became a physician. I grew up in Brooklyn, New York, where I acquired my ultimate unique and apparently permanent accent blend. Apart from experiencing a few cultural and educational challenges and adjustments in my new home environment early on, my assimilation into mainstream society proceeded smoothly. In fact, my progress accelerated during high school and my academic and athletic achievements enabled me to go on to college and then to medical school on scholarships.

Coincidentally, 1969 was the year my father died, at age sixty-nine, back in my village of Kalloni (which means *beauty*). I barely knew my father. My parents separated and then quickly divorced when I was six, and I only have vague recollections of our time together as a family before that time. My mother was thirty-two years old, and my father was twenty years her senior. They had been married for sixteen years.

In the middle of a day just prior to Christmas 1951, my mother suddenly plucked me out of school and transported me directly to Athens. My sister was sent to live with a maternal aunt in the city of Volos, and my brother remained with our father in Kalloni. I did not see my two older siblings until six years later; I briefly met up with them in 1957, just before they embarked on a ship sailing from Piraeus to New York City.

While in Athens, my mother and I endured many hardships,

mainly because of extreme poverty that was prevalent in post-World War II Athens. We shared a two-room home belonging to my maternal grandmother together with her two sons and her elderly half-sister, Aunt Elpiniki. My grandmother was also divorced. She possessed many extraordinary character traits. She was my hero, the unquestionable matriarch and pillar of strength that kept our family together and safe. She had a great work ethic and was a magician when it came to stretching every penny. Despite her meager salary as janitor at the dormitory of the ancient University of Athens, my grandmother managed to house and feed all of us, as well as to put two of her sons through the university that employed her. My mother also worked with her and contributed to the household expenses, cooking, cleaning and other duties. Both would frequently save the bus fare by walking the long distance to and from work. My mother had no social life, and over the next few years, I was often aware of her despair and heard her sobs in the night. I placed all the blame for the divorce and our misfortune on my father and harbored bitterness and resentment toward him that persisted and grew through my late teenage years.

In the meantime, my mother succeeded in obtaining a sponsored visa and immigrated to the United States in 1956; after remarrying— this time to a Greek man with U.S. citizenship—she became a naturalized citizen. This enabled her to obtain visas for my two older siblings in June 1958. I then left the protective umbrella of my grandmother and joined my mother and my siblings in the States in June 1959.

Just before my departure for America, my father traveled to Athens to wish me well and to say his goodbyes—it turned out to be the last time I saw him alive. I had not seen him for seven years. He became tearful while I remained stoic, and I interpreted his reaction as an admission of his guilt, as validation for my antipathy, even anger, toward him. As I matured, I pieced together more details about my father and the circumstances of the divorce, which challenged what I thought I knew about him. I became aware of his abundant love for my siblings and me. My father was highly admired by his community for his generosity, intellect, and command of the Greek language. During college, I established a regular correspondence with him, and he was proud to learn that all three of his children were accomplished, successful, and happy, and he took great pleasure in our achievements. After all, I became a physician, my brother managed a large and very popular restaurant in Brooklyn called the Golden Ox, and my sister owned her own beauty salon. But I could sense that my father was lonely without any of his children by his side, which made me feel ashamed and remorseful for having resented him so much the last time we met.

My father had been a chain smoker since childhood, and he died in December 1969 from emphysema compounded by pneumonia. During his illness, an aunt of mine in Kalloni cared for him. I was twenty-three years old, and when I received the news and realized how my father must have felt those last few days of his life, how he'd longed to have his children by his side, I broke down in tears. Though I reasoned that I could not have interrupted my medical school education and that I could not have afforded a trip to Greece, I still felt that my excuses for not being there for him were unsettling. When I was thirty-five, my wife and our two young daughters and I eventually travelled to Greece and visited his grave.

My parent's divorce had great influence on my character development. It caused me to become more self-reliant and to take responsibility for my own actions. This strengthened my determination to succeed as to be of help to my mother. My false impression of my father, taught me to consider the possibility that my judgment of others may sometimes be wrong which, in turn, made me introspective and, hence, more considerate of other people's opinions and perspectives.

To help enforce the Civil Rights Act of 1964, starting in 1969, the federal government mandated that 10 percent of an entering class at universities must consist of blacks and other minorities. Being Caucasian, integrated in main stream of society, and with good grades, I did not suspect that this affirmative action policy played a role in my personal acceptance to UB; I was simply grateful to have this opportunity.

This policy was challenged but generally upheld by the Bakke decision in 1978, when the U.S. Supreme Court argued that promoting minority student matriculation in medical school was justified on the basis of two main principles: 1, diversity of the student body promoted equality that benefited society at large, and 2, assuming that they would return and practice medicine in their underserved communities, these physicians would be more effective than Caucasians in forging a strong doctor-patient relationship and trust that could then translate into more effective patient care. (http://journalofethics.ama-assn. org/2012/12/hlaw1-1212.html; http://aamcdiversityfactsandfigures2016. org/report-section/section-3/)

In my opinion, the minority students adjusted well to the rigors of medical school. There was one exception, however, that I recall vividly. From the very start of a psychiatry class during my freshman year, an older black student struggled with the medical school curriculum. Our teacher, who I'll refer to as GLR, was knowledgeable, pleasant, and well liked. Because she was independently wealthy, she volunteered at the medical school. GLR often conducted her lectures at her home and served us a welcome free lunch. At one lecture during the second half of the year, this particular student suddenly stood up and went on a continuous ten-minute tirade, showering the professor with every known expletive, calling her white trash and other names. I was shocked. To this day, I cannot state with any certainty if this eruption was premeditated, spontaneous, or justified by reasons unknown to me. It was a sign of the times in our changing history. The student was dismissed the following week.

Upon completion of their medical training, many of the minority students pursued clinical practice outside of socially depressed or underserved areas. Thus, several geographic and ethnic health care disparities were not remedied by the Bakke decision. Regrettably, while trends indicate that application and enrollment to medical schools has increased, matriculation among black Americans has remained low and steady at about 6 percent (see statistics from 2015, https://academic.

). When interviewed, black American students contend that insufficient exposure to suitable role models is a central reason for this continuing trend. In contrast, matriculation of females, Hispanics, Asian Americans, and other ethnic groups has risen dramatically.

The year 1969 was eventful, even tumultuous, for our nation. Richard Nixon was inaugurated president and begun to de-escalate the very unpopular Vietnam War. Young men were injured or died by the hundreds of thousands, triggering angry and violent protests across the United States. At that time, the draft was still in effect. Ways to evade the draft included serving in the National Guard or Reserve Officers' Training Corps (ROTC) program, being married with children, or enrolling in a college or university, which explains why about 75 percent of draftees were socioeconomically disadvantaged. Many large-scale protests against the U.S. invasion of Cambodia took place at colleges and universities. These protests were somewhat ironic, since most of the protestors were students who could legally avoid being drafted. Morally, however, I was one of many students who was conflicted, experiencing guilt and other negative feelings at seeing other young men die while I was safe and pursuing my medical studies and a promising future.

The year 1969 was also memorable in several other respects. For the first time, I witnessed the blatant and egregious use of drugs at the school campus. Drugs, sex and rock-and -roll, were also celebrated at Woodstock at Bethel, New York where 400,000 people partied that summer. It was also the year that Neil Armstrong and Edwin "Buzz" Aldrin became the first man to walk on the moon, that the Charles Manson murders took place, and that the violent Stonewall Riot in New York City came to symbolize the start of the gay rights movement in the United States.

WHY A NEPHROLOGY CAREER?

―――――⚬⚬⚬―――――

INFLUENCE OF MY TEACHERS IN MEDICAL SCHOOL

I AM NOT a firm believer in the concept of destiny, but from the very start, my pediatric nephrology career seemed inevitable. When I entered medical school, like most of my classmates, I was an enthusiastic and impressionable neophyte, and the cards were heavily stacked in favor of nephrology for me, almost to the exclusion of other medical specialties. Let me explain why?

In the late 1960s, UB was on the cutting edge of renal pathology research. This became possible because two renowned scientists at UB, Dr. Felix Milgnom, an immunologist, and Dr. Giuseppe Andres, a nephropathologist, were joined by a younger but very ambitious and dynamic pathologist from Harvard, Dr. Robert T. McCluskey. Dr. McCluskey was very interested in the immunologic basis of acquired renal disorders and reasoned that collaboration between top leaders from several scientific disciplines could accelerate common research interests, much as translational research or program grants today serve as catalysts for research focused on specific disorders. These same individuals taught my general pathology course, and their enthusiasm for nephropathology was infectious. In addition, several outstanding clinical nephrologists in Buffalo served as role models away from the classroom. They were exceptional in applying basic science information to explain challenging kidney disorders of their patients. Then, when I witnessed the successful use of steroids to manage two children who presented with nephrotic syndrome (NS) and anasarca (severe total body swelling), I became convinced that they could perform miracles.

With this prelude, it is not surprising that I was "pre-programmed" to pursue nephrology as my career objective. Apparently, I was not the only one who was inspired by these pioneers and great mentors of nephrology. As I discovered a few years later, a staggering 10% of my entire graduating class went on to become adult nephrologists.

REYES SYNDROME TRAGEDY

My choice to enter the pediatric nephrology specialty became solidified during my pediatric internship and residency training at Children's Hospital of Pittsburgh. I was personally involved in the care of twelve children during the Reye's syndrome epidemic of 1973 and 1974. Nearly all of the children were previously healthy except for recent viral symptoms that progressed to include severe vomiting, mental confusion, lethargy or coma, and rapid breathing. The neurologic symptoms were induced by brain swelling caused by an acid blood pH and high blood ammonia levels associated with an acutely enlarged and poorly functioning liver. Most children died despite receiving what may now be viewed as a primitive and ineffective form of manual peritoneal dialysis to lower the ammonia levels. This condition was later linked to use of salicylate or aspirin-containing products to manage certain viral disorders such as influenza, "flu," or chickenpox. The exact pathophysiology of the condition remains enigmatic to this day, but it is largely preventable nowadays because pediatricians warn against the use of aspirin during the flu season. I conjectured that if we only had more effective dialysis or hemoperfusion capability—passing large volumes of blood through an adsorbent substance—to remove ammonia and allow time for the acute liver disorder to resolve, we could save the lives of these children and avoid the immense grief experienced by the families and by the helpless hospital staff. Pursuing nephrology could impart training on these techniques and thus enable me to accomplish this goal.

Other considerations contributed to my decision to enter the nephrology field. It was abundantly clear to me from the start that I had no talent for business and that administering a private pediatric practice—with hiring personnel, payroll and billing responsibilities—was of little interest to me. Moreover, I was fascinated by a variety of complex clinical disorders and the only way I could sustain my intellectual stimulation was to remain in academic medicine within pediatrics. In addition, I welcomed the opportunity to teach and do research. After considerable thought about what specialty was the most encompassing, I came to the inescapable conclusion that pediatric nephrology met all my requirements. After forty years in this field, I can categorically state that pediatric nephrology far surpassed all my expectations.

Pediatric training at Children's Hospital of Pittsburgh (CHP): Patients always come first

～⌘～

BEFORE I COULD embark on a nephrology career, I was most fortunate to have my pediatric residency training at CHP. I was privileged to have awesome and legendary mentors in pediatrics, such as Drs. Paul Gaffney, Tim Oliver, and Jack Paradise, among others. I also developed immense respect for CHP as an institution and all the people that are part of the CHP family. Long before we had the present amazing CHP facility, at that time patients were housed in small, eight-by-ten-foot rooms in the 125-year-old building. However, CHP was always special because of the staff's genuine love and devotion in caring for sick children and their families. This was not only noticeable in the actions of doctors and nurses, but extended to janitors, hospital telephone operators, laboratory personnel, pharmacists, medical records employees, security guards, parking attendants, and all other workers. The special, personal touch readily evident at CHP was not as impressive in several other institutions where I trained—in my opinion, this is still the single most important factor accounting for the exceptional patient outcomes at CHP. I was so impressed and inspired by this aspect that after completing my nephrology fellowship, I was most eager

11

to return to Pittsburgh, my home by choice, to join this great team of caregivers. I believe that the following anecdote personifies the team spirit prevailing at CHP at the time of my second year of residency training in 1974.

GIOVANNI AND HIS VERY SPECIAL MOM

THIS EVENT TOOK place at around two o'clock in the morning. I was especially busy that night. I was in the process of admitting a very sick child, and while passing through a patient ward, I heard a child whimpering through the partly open door of his otherwise dark room. I walked in and found an eight-year-old boy with a large, protruding abdomen sitting on the side of the bed, copious tears rolling down his cheeks. After asking why he cried and if he was hurting, in a syncopated, tearful voice he replied, "I'm not hurting, but I'm scared I'll die; I want my mommy." I was not personally familiar with him or his medical condition, yet I assured him that everything was going to be OK. I promised that once I finished my admission, I would return to see him.

After completing my admission, I reviewed the medical chart before going back to visit the boy, and discovered that he had an inoperable, malignant tumor in his liver. I then entered his now quiet room and found him content and in the arms of a woman who worked as a night janitor. She had done a wonderful job in calming him down. I thanked her for taking the initiative to be a surrogate mother for this unfortunate child in his hour of need. I recognized this woman as one of four women of Italian ethnicity who worked diligently as a team to keep the floors of our then-ancient hospital in meticulous, spic-and-span shape. I had previously witnessed situations when these women acted outside the limits of their work description as dictated by the circumstances, guided by their maternal instincts and by their conscience. These women epitomized the work ethic and deep-rooted human values that had so impressed me and forged my very favorable opinion of Pittsburgh and its inhabitants. Sadly, the boy died a week later.

About four years later, after returning to CHP as a staff physician, I met a young man in his early twenties while playing soccer at Schenley Park. His name was Giovanni. He was a good player and seemed to enjoy being on my pick-up team on several occasions throughout that summer. Despite the difference in our ages, we became friends on the soccer field. To my surprise, while I was rounding one Saturday afternoon, I saw Giovanni at CHP wearing a blue hospital-issued volunteer shirt. I smiled in surprise and asked what he was doing there. He said that he had been a volunteer at CHP for three years and very much enjoyed spending time there. I noticed that he had the same last name on his ID tag as the Italian woman that I had met on the night mentioned above four years earlier. She was his mom. I related to him the above incident and endorsed that his mother and people like her had influenced my decision to return to Pittsburgh and CHP. In conversing with him, he informed me that he would be completing his college education a year later and hoped to matriculate in medical school upon graduation. He guardedly asked me for a recommendation letter to include with his medical school applications and appeared surprised that I accepted so quickly. Of course, I wrote a very positive letter on his behalf and told him that I did this primarily out of my gratitude and great respect for his mother. I also shared with him that my own mother, whom I loved and respected immensely, at one time was a janitor at the dormitories at the University of Athens, Greece, when I was in grammar school. After graduating from Temple University Giovanni went on to become a very fine surgeon and I am quite certain that he took excellent and well-deserved care of his mom.

Start of my nephrology fellowship at Children's Hospital National Medical Center (chnmc), in Washington DC

WITH THE ABOVE brief background, you can appreciate why I eagerly anticipated an exciting career in pediatric nephrology. Indeed, my fellowship experience supplied me with a much broader perspective of the general field of nephrology and of the more challenging issues facing children per se. What I did not foresee, however, is that the very first day of my nephrology fellowship at CHNMC would start with a bang.

I was in the process of receiving an orientation of the hospital, conducted by my pediatric nephrology chief, Dr. James Chan. When we approached the ICU, he informed me that our service was requested to perform a new consult at that unit— a one-day-old baby with anasarca (generalized body edema or swelling) and massive proteinuria (high urinary losses of protein). Upon entering the ICU, we encountered a large group of physicians actively resuscitating a newborn. It turned out to be our consult. All resuscitation efforts failed, and the baby died. I learned that the mother was a prostitute who worked at a nearby 16th-Street location. She refused an autopsy on her baby but consented to a less-invasive kidney biopsy while the baby's body was still in the ICU.

Dr. Chan turned to me and said, "Since there is no risk to the patient, this is an ideal situation for you to practice performing a percutaneous renal biopsy." This procedure had just become possible to perform at the bedside because of the advent of a special biopsy needle (Tru-Cut) and by the clinical use of a novel, noninvasive technique called *ultrasonography*, which we used to localize the lower pole of the kidney. Prior to that time, because of a high risk of bleeding associated with percutaneous renal biopsies especially in children, biopsies were rare and mainly performed surgically under direct visualization of the kidney in an operating room, with the patient under general anesthesia. These factors rendered kidney biopsies cumbersome and expensive.

On the day following what appeared to be a technically well-done biopsy of this baby, I was urgently informed by the pathology service that spirochetes were visible in the renal biopsy tissue; these were also found on nasal swab specimens. This proved that death was caused by disseminated syphilis, which also explained the associated congenital nephrotic syndrome and anasarca. As a result, over fifty caretakers who had contact or were involved in the resuscitation process were advised to receive a large penicillin dosage injected deep into the buttocks. Where does a budding nephrologist go from this unique case? Well, I assure you that I had many other interesting patient encounters at CHNMC and throughout my career.

One of the most notable aspects of my fellowship, was my association with Gregory Buffone, Ph.D. Greg was a young, energetic, and capable scientist who headed the very busy Clinical Laboratory at CHNMC. His main research interest revolved around the quantitation of blood proteins of clinical relevance using a variety of new techniques, such as immunodiffusion in agar plates and "rocket" methods. I was aware of his research focus before seeking him out. Greg immediately showed enthusiasm at the prospect of collaborating with me on a clinical research project to measure urinary proteins utilizing urine specimens from our renal patients that were sent to the main clinical laboratory for routine purposes. He allocated a small space in his lab, helped me set up, and supervised my research project. My work led to the publication of a new method for measuring urinary albumin even when present in very small quantities, or *microalbuminuria*, which I hypothesized to be an early marker of the subsequent development of more serious or overt renal disease. This was born out of the fact that, like most pediatricians, I was primed to think more along the lines of disease prevention than treatment. As I discuss later in this book under "*Research, Sub-specialization*" and "*Diabetes and the fabulous nephelometer*", this collaboration with Greg led to the development of a prototype instrument (Hyland nephelometer) to measure microalbuminuria. This seemingly minor research project was fortuitous and led to an unanticipated, large pay-off during my academic career (see p.142).

The 1960s and 1970s were a dynamic, historic, and transformative period for the specialty of pediatric nephrology. In my view, two major reasons account for this transformation: one, the International Study of Kidney Diseases in Children (ISKDC) and two, the emergence of dialysis/renal transplantation on a large scale.

There is little doubt that pediatric nephrology established its distinct identity in conjunction with the landmark ISKDC study that was conceived by Drs. Henry Barnett and Chester Edelman in 1965 and was realized from 1967 to 1974. This was preceded by the biopsy confirmation and classification of several glomerular disorders of children mainly during the early 1960s. These diverse disorders were previously included under a single clinical diagnosis known as *Bright's disease*. That term was coined since Sir Richard Bright's initial publication in 1825 of children who developed dark or bloody urine after tonsillar infection and was finally abandoned largely because of the ISKDC findings. Once there was agreement on the different renal conditions based on the biopsy appearance or morphologic classification, the need for establishing clinicopathologic correlations—including clinical symptoms and signs and response to treatment—became apparent. Apart from providing uniform guidelines for treatment of the various glomerular disorders and determining their long-term outcome, the ISKDC illustrated the solidarity and common purpose of pediatric nephrologists from all over the world and tested their resolve to organize a study of unprecedented magnitude. In fact, adult nephrologists subsequently emulated the paradigm of the pediatric nephrologists by conducting similar multi-center trials. In my opinion, the ISKDC deserves the credit for the emergence of the American Society of Pediatric Nephrology in 1976 and the American Society of Nephrology in 1979. Also, the publication of several new journals devoted to pediatric nephrology dovetailed with the ISKDC. These journals represented an important platform for focused awareness and research of renal disorders relevant to children. Prior to the SKIDC, scientific contributions by pediatric nephrologists were published in general pediatric or adult journals, such as Dr. Shalhoub's hypothesis on the immunologic basis of nephrotic syndrome, which was published in the *Lancet* in 1975. The ISKDC study also sparked the development of new methods of direct immunologic testing utilizing biopsy tissue, including an evaluation of multiple components of the complement pathway, a part of the immune system that plays a key role in the pathogenesis of glomerulonephritis. This progress encouraged subsequent discoveries and testing of novel biomarkers of renal disease, such as anti-neutrophilic antibodies (ANCA), immune complexes, and, more recently, genetic testing for podocytopathies utilizing blood samples.

Many readers may be surprised to learn that prior to the availability of life-sustaining dialysis, the pediatric nephrology field attracted relatively few, but very eclectic, dedicated scholarly physicians and researchers. These individuals were mainly intrigued by the kidney's avant-garde physiology that came to the forefront in the 1940s and 1950s through the efforts of several world-renowned physiologists, such as Homer W. Smith. These talented and charismatic researchers established that the central role of the kidney was to regulate blood pressure through control of body fluids and electrolytes, as well as describe diabetic nephropathy and several other fascinating and important but largely untreatable disorders. This relatively limited scope of nephrology changed drastically and rapidly in the early 1970's because of the emergence of dialysis and renal transplantation as viable treatment options for chronic or end-stage renal failure.

By 1972, the cause of many glomerular, hypertensive, and congenital renal disorders remained poorly understood, had no remedy, and were inexorably progressive and often lethal. This dismal outlook completely changed in October 1972, when the United States Congress approved Law 92-603, which authorized funding for the end-stage renal disease (ESRD) Program under Medicare. This landmark law entitled individuals with ESRD to receive dialysis and/or renal transplantation with all medical payments underwritten by Medicare, regardless of their income. These treatment modalities together with several other medical breakthroughs that followed, gave hope for a more meaningful long-term patient survival. As a result, the number of Americans receiving dialysis rose exponentially, and dialysis was no longer limited to patients with acute or reversible kidney failure or wealthy individuals who could afford chronic dialysis services. This single law spawned a multibillion-dollar industry including dialysis facilities, nursing and technical personnel, equipment, and ESRD-related medications. Progress with renal transplantation followed but lagged behind dialysis because of the low efficacy and safety concerns associated with the existing monolithic steroid/azathioprine immunosuppressive regimen. As I note later in the book, the availability of cyclosporine and the pioneering work here at the University Health Center of Pittsburgh starting in May 1981 dramatically changed the transplantation landscape.

GRADUATION FROM FELLOWSHIP

COINCIDING WITH PASSAGE of Public Law 92-603 in 1972 came the first board examination that qualified a physician to become a "nephrology specialist" and not just a pediatrician or an internist with special interest in electrolytes, acid-base balance, and edematous—body swelling—disorders related to derangements in plasma aldosterone and natriuretic peptides. To get this special designation, in addition to passing a written examination—which is the main requirement today—one had to also pass an oral examination. The latter required me to face directly two preeminent pediatric nephrologists who had come to Washington, D.C., expressly to examine me. They presented me with two clinical case scenarios, each of which I had to discuss over a forty-five-minute period. After being permitted to ask additional questions about the medical history, physical exam, and laboratory values, I was expected to prioritize the possible diagnoses, request further evaluation, and offer a management plan. After arriving at the most likely diagnosis, one of the examiners asked me, "What other conditions would you consider?" "None", I replied with confidence, but after I left the small examination room, I felt very insecure and was pessimistic about having passed this test.

Fortunately, I did pass on the first try, but I recall how stressful this was. Because of lack of uniformity in administering such oral tests, as well as the considerable expense incurred by the trainees, the practice was later abandoned. Only two years later, I had the pleasure of interacting with my celebrated interviewers as a colleague. Both made significant research contributions and are now considered founding members of pediatric nephrology. At the young age of thirty-one, Dr. Jack Metcoff had organized the first conference devoted exclusively to nephrotic syndrome in 1948 (he died at seventy-seven, in 1994). And Dr. Warren E. Grupe from Boston Children's Hospital successfully utilized chlorambucil and steroids as immunomodulators in the management of minimal change disease or lipoid nephrosis.

While my fellowship training was very effective from the clinical perspective, it did not prepare me for the mission I was about to undertake—establish and manage a brand-new nephrology program at a major university-based pediatric hospital (see below). The challenge was at once exciting and scary, but the prospect of paving my own future was compelling and, frankly, irresistible. Though it was implicit, I did not once consider how daunting this task would be without the support of other nephrology colleagues with whom I could discuss challenging cases, exchange ideas, and share night and weekend call. As things turned out, at first, I did not even have the luxury of turning the service over to a non-nephrology colleague as to allow me to take vacation with my family without experiencing guilt over endangering the welfare of children under my care.

Major issues confronting children
with chronic renal failure
at the start of my nephrology career

Despite the affordability of dialysis and transplantation made possible by Law 92-603, it became quickly apparent that most pediatric hospitals were slow in responding to the needs of children with ESRD. There were insufficient numbers of nephrologists, personnel with experience in pediatric dialysis, or dedicated nephrology clinics and services. In addition, partly because of the urgency to manage the huge backlog of adults with ESRD, industry delayed addressing the dialysis-related equipment needs of children. Thus, dialysis-related issues posed the most important impediment to the short-term survival of children with ESRD during the 1970s and 1980s. Renal transplantation, which is widely considered to be the only acceptable means for achieving long-term meaningful survival in children, was also hampered mainly because of ineffective and toxic immunosuppression medications and less so by the need of special surgical techniques.

I was most fortunate to have my nephrology training at Children's Hospital National Medical Center (CHNMC) in Washington, D.C. This was one of a handful of pediatric hospitals in the United States that had started a full-scale chronic hemodialysis program in 1973.

My exposure to this program enabled me to learn a great deal about this life-saving but labor-intensive process of blood purification across a commercially available, semipermeable membrane. One of the main obstacles to chronic hemodialysis in the pediatric population was the creation of vascular access. The long-term viability of such access depended on the development of new surgical techniques, biocompatible materials, tube sizes suitable for smaller children, and preventing or overcoming exit site and systemic infections. Another obstacle was the unavailability of both suitable dialysis machines and dialyzers requiring low blood volume for priming as not to cause a major fall in blood pressure when employed in infants and younger children. In addition, because there were so few centers that performed chronic dialysis in younger children, this life-saving modality was only available to families residing in proximity to pediatric hospitals having a dialysis unit. Even if a local outpatient dialysis unit was willing to accept an older child for dialysis, because of competition for the limited hemodialysis slots, these treatments were often scheduled at odd hours of the day such as from 8:00 p.m. to midnight. This had a negative impact on the child's sleep, energy level and school performance and was disruptive to the lifestyle of the entire family. Moreover, such children were exposed to psychological trauma because they were dialyzed adjacent to elderly adults experiencing medical emergencies while dialyzing. Also, because demand for dialysis exceeded the available resources, adults with diabetes or lupus were initially excluded from treatment because they were gauged as having poor long-term outlook. Similarly, children with superimposed medical or cognitive conditions, birth defects, or those deemed to have inadequate family financial or educational resources were often unjustly denied this life-sustaining modality.

New procedures and basic safety guidelines for dialyzing infants and younger children had to be developed. Pediatric nephrology and dialysis staff had to be trained. Hospital facilities had to become compliant with extensive government regulations. I was confronted with these challenging issues immediately after I took charge of the nascent Division of Nephrology at CHP, right after my renal fellowship. In addition, there were no vascular or other surgeons at CHP who were familiar with the various peritoneal or subclavian dialysis catheters or how to insert them. Hence, I had to devise my own complete sterilized sets that included trocars and catheters, gauze, syringes, and needles, all wrapped up in green-colored sterilizable (or autoclavable) cloth. My skill in inserting these catheters gradually improved but eventually I was glad and relieved to relinquish these procedures to a most capable young surgeon, Dr. Eugene Weiner. Incidentally, I also assembled my own renal biopsy sets and performed all renal biopsies.

Although the nationally funded dialysis program grew rapidly, renal transplantation lagged well behind and could not accommodate the large number of patients with ESRD awaiting transplantation. This disparity is largely explained by the delay in discovery of more efficacious immunosuppressive agents until much later, in 1981, and because there were insufficient organ donors to meet the demand.

Funding of care for the large number of existing patients with chronic kidney failure was a major catalyst for the overall growth of the nephrology field and gave rise to the very lucrative medical and dialysis industries. Lobbyists linked to the new dialysis industry were promoting the interests of their employers by influencing politicians while sales personnel were ubiquitous at hospitals, national conferences, and other venues where they could enhance sales of their products. Dialysis and pharmaceutical companies sponsored national nephrology symposia as well as smaller gatherings to promote their products on hospital premises, often granting honoraria to speakers and providing elaborate dinners and other amenities to attract attendees. They also sponsored bona fide academic educational and research opportunities. For example, the application and funding of the North American Pediatric Renal Transplant Cooperative Study (NAPRTCS) was declined by governmental agencies and was made possible only because of the generous sponsorship of Sandoz, the large pharmaceutical company and purveyor of the anti-rejection drug, cyclosporine. This led to several important studies that were of benefit to children.

It is worth stressing, however, that the interdependence between industry and nephrologists crossed ethical boundaries and, on occasion, may well have been detrimental to patient care. An obvious example of such conflict of interest occurred in the early 1990s and involved NAPRTCS and one of its most prominent and influential leaders. Although the methodology and contributions of NAPRTCS were laudable, this preeminent leader had repeatedly voiced harsh and unfounded criticisms against a newer competitor of cyclosporine, tacrolimus. His remarks at national meetings favored the ongoing use of cyclosporine, thereby benefitting its marketer, the sponsor of NAPRTCS, Sandoz. This obvious conflict of interest persisted well after several credible studies, including our own data, had demonstrated that tacrolimus was a superior immunosuppressive agent (Comparison of FK-506 and cyclosporine regimens in pediatric renal transplantation. Pediatr Nephrol 8(2):193-200, 1994; Clinical use of tacrolimus (FK-506) in infants and children with renal transplants. Pediatr Nephrol 9:487-494, 1995; Current expectations in pediatric renal transplantation. Current Opin in Organ Transplant 1:37-43, 1996). This action likely delayed the use –and benefit– of tacrolimus in the general pediatric transplant population for several years, until the evidence eventually became irrefutable.

In addition, a variety of products were promoted without adequate demonstration of their superiority compared to less expensive products. As a result, the cost of ESRD care exploded until legislation was enacted to curb these costs; currently, dialysis in the United States costs about $90,000 per person per year and the total cost of this program exceeds $35 billion a year. To avert such conflicts of interest, hospitals now ban any sales pitches on their premises. In addition, the Physician Payments Sunshine Act passed in 2013 requires drug and medical device makers to disclose payments or gifts made to doctors and teaching hospitals. The explicit aim of this law is to educate patients about conflicts of interest arising when drug companies support medical research, education, and clinical decisions that ultimately lead to an unfair market advantage. However, many corporations have found innovative alternative means for promoting sales of their health care products, such as heavy advertising directly to the consumer through standard media or by lobbying politicians to raise Medicare payments related to dialysis.

Even though pediatric dialysis services became increasingly available at most pediatric hospitals during the 1970s, the results for long-term survival and quality of life remained suboptimal, especially in infants and younger children. As a result, several well-meaning pediatric psychologists and psychiatrists, as well as budding medical bioethicists, opposed the performance of chronic dialysis or transplantation in younger infants and children. One of the senior psychiatrists at CHP, Dr. John "Jack" Reinhart, had published an editorial in 1970 in which he questioned the appropriateness of this approach to what was then considered a uniformly fatal condition. He wrote, "I seriously question the value of chronic dialysis or renal transplant. Despite the physician's desire to heal and parents' willingness for 'anything to be done,' I feel that programs of dialysis and renal transplants for children should be carefully evaluated, not in terms of gross survival, but in parameters of meaningful growth and development living. We may find the price the child pays for life too great at present" (Reinhart JB. The doctor's dilemma; whether to recommend continuous renal dialysis or renal homotransplantations for the child with end-stage renal disease. *J. Pediatr.* 1970; 77:505–507).

Even though I was young, ambitious, enthusiastic, and confident in my abilities when I first joined the CHP staff in 1977, I had to overcome this still-prevailing oppositional mind-set of my older, highly respected and influential colleagues. To succeed in this task, I first had to convince them that I could lead a team capable of achieving good outcomes in this high-risk population. This goal was most daunting given the scarcity of trained pediatric dialysis nurses and technical personnel who could assist me.

Despite the clear ethical and logistical concerns, more and more centers began to offer dialysis to infants. With perseverance, dedication, diligence, and increased clinical experience, outcomes greatly improved.

Return to Children's Hospital of Pittsburgh (CHP)

A FEW MONTHS before graduating from my fellowship program in Washington, D.C., I received a telephone call from the chairman of pediatrics at CHP, Dr. T. K. Oliver, who was a great mentor and friend throughout my residency training. Apparently, he had followed my career closely, and after making inquiries about my performance from my fellowship program director, Dr. James Chan, he offered me a job—without an interview or any discussion of contract, salary, or other employment conditions. I can still recall Dr. Oliver's exact words during his brief but important telephone call that determined my career path and my family's future: "Demetri, don't bother looking for another job; we need you to return to Pittsburgh and establish a first-class nephrology program." This was a most enticing offer from a man whom I very much admired and respected both for his superior intellect and his personal and professional qualities. I was also grateful to him for accepting me so generously into his residency program and for contributing to my professional development. I had received another much more lucrative job offer at another hospital in Pennsylvania, but the promise of academic growth and the overall opportunity available at CHP was far superior. My wife and I were also attracted to Pittsburgh for the lifestyle and educational opportunities that we wished for our two young daughters, as well as the work prospects for my wife as an education specialist. Thus, we both quickly decided to accept the position in Pittsburgh. It was an important step for us, and we never looked back or regretted this decision.

Beginning of my academic
nephrology career at CHP

When I first joined the CHP staff in 1977, there were a total of thirty-five staff physicians, five administrators, and several secretarial and other ancillary personnel. I was already well acquainted with the physicians from my extensive interaction with them during residency training, which made my professional transition to CHP easier, since I was immediately and warmly accepted and supported. I was also familiar with the administrators, one of whom was a tennis partner of mine and later became CEO of CHP. Because CHP was affiliated with the University of Pittsburgh, School of Medicine, my official employer was the University of Pittsburgh. Therefore, my full initial title was: Demetrius Ellis, M.D., Director of Pediatric Nephrology at CHP, Assistant Professor of Pediatrics and Nephrology, University of Pittsburgh School of Medicine.

I was so enamored by this impressive title that I gave no thought to the length of my work day or how low my salary scale was. My wife, Irene, made sure that our children were well taken care of, so I felt less guilty about spending so much time away from home. This meant that Irene had to stop teaching and that we had to live under moderately strict budgetary constraints. My salary was limited as per my contract and was frozen for nearly five years; there was no additional compensation for overtime and no bonuses were given based on my rapidly increasing clinical productivity and billing. As strange as it may seem, my starting salary was only marginally higher than that of a high school graduate employed as an inexperienced union worker at a steel mill factory in Pittsburgh. The large salaries paid to these workers and little investment in more efficient technologies to produce steel made the United States less competitive with other nations and led to the eventual decline of this indispensable industry. Fortunately, the economy of Pittsburgh quickly bounced back in good measure because of the exceptional contributions by several of its universities that were at the cutting edge of the technologic and medical revolutions.

Career Overview

My personal clinical experience is not only extensive but also unique. First, starting as a single practitioner of nephrology in a busy academic hospital, I invested eighty to ninety hours per week, including weekend and night call, and had forty-two years of uninterrupted clinical contact with patients. This was made possible by my great enjoyment of my work. I invested a substantial portion of my time in keeping current in my field through extensive reading of numerous scientific articles that I filed under a system of my own design. My clinical acumen was enhanced by attending and also by delivering numerous lectures devoted to challenging patients as well as an array of thought-provoking renal topics. Also, practicing nephrology at a major pediatric center that treated nearly all children with renal disorders for a hundred-mile referral radius assured a heavy caseload but also a great variety of clinical disorders. My experience was further enriched by the fact that I maintained metrics on interventions and clinical outcomes in children with specific clinical disorders, which I then subjected to rigorous statistical analysis with the eventual aim of sharing or publishing the results in reputable pediatric medical journals. To accomplish this goal requires a thorough review of the existing medical literature, which was extremely time-consuming, particularly in the pre-internet era, so I could have a complete foundation for making critical comparisons of my patient outcome results to those of other investigators. This process was tremendously instructive, as it induced me to read scientific articles much more carefully and critically. Furthermore, I received feedback and positive reinforcement of my own research conclusions by way of expert journal reviewers and editors and from nephrology colleagues who attended my research presentations at various scientific venues. As an editor and reviewer of articles for several journals, I also had opportunity to critically review the work of other investigators seeking publication of their own articles. Employing these disciplines helped to sharpen my own analytical skills and scientific writing.

Because of my substantial clinical workload right from the inception of my professional career, as well as my personal aversion to politics, committee duties, and administrative work, I declined several invitations to accept positions on pediatric nephrology organizations, societies and journal editorial boards. For similar reasons, I later declined offers that could have accelerated my career by way of accepting coveted high-level academic pediatric leadership positions, such as chairman of pediatrics at various academic institutions or journal editor-in-chief. I was convinced that my personal talents and personality traits were much more suitable for hands-on clinical nephrology and that I would be happier, and ultimately more effective, by focusing on this endeavor. In essence, I aspired to do what I did best. I hasten to add, however, that I deeply appreciate the efforts of many of my nephrology colleagues who organized and led educational symposia that stimulated clinical and translational research and disseminated such information. These individuals, who promoted education free of personal bias and independently of outside interests or influences, deserve my personal gratitude as well as all the accolades and awards conferred on them by various organizations. In contrast, my preferred means for contributing to the advancement of nephrology was through a discipline of active and sustained dissemination of clinical research and review articles. This process not only promoted my personal education and fulfilled my need to remain current with an ever- expanding body of medical information, but, in the process, it also continued to fuel my enthusiasm for a broad range of nephrology topics. The net effect and objective of all of these efforts was simply to improve the care and quality of life of the children and families under my care. Indeed, I aspired to achieve the highest level of expertise in my field and deliver medical care in a humane manner, guided by knowledge but also a good measure of common sense, with the child's welfare always being the utmost priority. In doing so, I hoped to become a role model for younger physicians, as others had been for me—this is my professional legacy. First and foremost, this is reflected by the emotions and feedback expressed in the letters sent to me by the children and families that I treated. In addition, my legacy is evident in the gloating evaluations I received for teaching of medical students, residents, and renal fellows with whom I had the privilege of interacting for well over four decades. Finally, the recognition and awards I received for my research, other scholarly activities and leadership contributions, are the icing on the cake.

I have worked hard throughout my life and have no regrets about that. However, sometimes I felt as though I was a juggler at a circus because I was constantly multitasking. By necessity, the interventions and outcomes of very ill children I managed in the ICU and hospital wards were under continuous scrutiny by many highly trained colleagues and coworkers. I was keenly aware that dropping the ball could have serious repercussions, principally for the patients but also for my personal reputation. This amount of responsibility caused brief periods of stress, usually several times during each day, as I pondered whether I had done everything possible to save a child or to avert a foreseeable catastrophe. Oddly enough, the vast majority of the time, I was so focused on my tasks that I lost all awareness of passing of time, the amount of work at hand, and even the medical complexity and challenges faced. In addition, it seemed that I gradually trained myself to endure, suppress, or delay satisfying thirst, hunger, or the need to attend to other bodily functions. Perhaps this became possible by the euphoria I experienced in witnessing my evaluations and plans come to successful fruition.

This raised my self-esteem and reinforced my confidence in making sound clinical decisions with subsequent patient encounters.

Of course, introspection also enabled me to be more objective in judging if my decisions were detrimental to my patients. If in hindsight, I was convinced that a different approach would not have had a superior outcome, I resolved not to experience prolonged psychological stress or remorse. Conversely, I was cognizant of the fact that, like other people, doctors are also fallible, and that accidents and miscalculations are not always avoidable. Under these circumstances, poor clinical outcomes are very painful and difficult to endure, even if, on balance, the physician's overall performance and results are consistently favorable. One hopes to learn from such experiences and apply this knowledge in improving future patient assessment and risk-benefit decisions. In summary, so long as I did not ruminate on my successes or failures, I found introspection to be a very constructive tool because it compelled me to think what steps I needed to take in order to learn, grow and progress in my decision-making process.

On a personal level, my commitment to my marriage and parenthood are of paramount importance. Based on the immeasurable amount of love that I have received from my wife and children over the years, I believe that I fare extremely high on this score. Faith is another element that is important to me. Religion has many benefits, including living life with an acute sense of conscience and peaceful coexistence and respect for my fellow man, while providing hope and giving a greater meaning to life here on earth. I am hopeful that God will judge me kindly. This is followed by my near obsession with sports and love of athletic competition, which had a very positive impact on other dimensions of my life. My numerous trophies tell only part of my sports legacy, which, by all accounts, has already inspired all three of our grandchildren. I freely admit that the order of these objectives may have been blurred from time to time. However, in general, I approached these simple but key objectives with effort, discipline, constant awareness, and self-reassessment.

What is "academic medicine"?

ACCORDING TO THE dictionary, *academic* is a noun referring to an educator at a college or university. It is also an adjective connoting a connection to "a narrow focus or display in learning especially in trivial aspects" or "hypothetical and theoretical pursuits which are not expected to produce an immediate or practical result." Although many medical specialists and especially pediatric nephrologists are employed by university-affiliated hospitals, their work can hardly be characterized as narrow focused, trivial, or impractical. In my view, *academic medicine* may be more broadly and simply defined as a dedication to teaching and scholarly activities applied under highly ethical guidelines with the ultimate goal of improving the health of those entrusted to our care.

For purposes of this book, the term *academic* denotes physicians who specialize in a particular field of medicine and receive a professorial rank from a medical school associated with a university or another acclaimed institution. In contrast to family physicians, internists and other doctors who are self-employed and are in greater control of setting the fees, hours, and general stipulations of their private practice, those employed in academic medicine have much less autonomy. They must work within the confines, rules, and obligations imposed by the medical school or institution that employs them. The latter includes accountability to the administrators who make sure that doctors remain in compliance with multiple regulatory agencies, billing for clinical services and various time deadlines; the chairman of the department who is their immediate boss; and the physician hierarchy within their specialty or division. This means that experiencing some stress is expected and, in truth, inevitable. Personally, I was only superficially familiar with most key duties expected of physicians in academic medicine described below, and I grossly underestimated the administrative workload, risks, and ramifications of being a division chief in a major academic institution.

While most academic physicians work at university-affiliated hospitals or facilities, they are actually employees of the university. The extent of direct patient care or clinical duties ranges from full-time to as little as one month per year, and the amount of time expended in administrative responsibilities, and/or "protected" time for research is also flexible or negotiable. The common thread is that nearly all specialists involved in academic medicine are expected to devote a major portion of time and effort on activities that do not directly generate revenue. These include education and scholarly activities that enhance the reputation of the physician and his/her employer, as well as participation on multiple committees that are essential to the function of the medical school and of the predominant facility at which they are assigned.

Above all else, physicians in academic medicine are educators. These professors at medical schools teach anatomy, pathology, physiology, pharmacology, and other basic sciences. These subjects form the backbone of medicine. Teaching is also a daily and intensive endeavor at university-affiliated hospitals in which students and residents undergo clinical training. Despite my heavy and continuous clinical load, I taught residents, renal fellows, and medical students on a daily basis throughout my career. My objective was to provide credible explanations of the medical conditions and their pathophysiology and thereby justify the medical decisions. This is an invaluable experience for those in training because it brings joy and also reinforces their confidence in their decision-making and their craft. To some extent, this ideology was also instilled in me when I was a student and medical trainee. I also presented formal lectures on renal topics of general pediatric interest, such as hypertension, proteinuria, urinary tract infections, and more. For students, review of these topics would prove handy later on when they were taking board examinations and applying for medical licensure. In addition, I participated in patient discussions and grand rounds lectures that placed me in direct contact with practicing pediatricians who also attended these conferences as part of their continuing medical education (CME). Such participation is required for medical license renewal and for determining eligibility to apply for medical malpractice insurance. Physicians employed in an academic capacity frequently, but not always, receive a salary that is determined on the basis of the median income of members of their specialty practicing in a specific geographic location in the United States; minor bonuses may be added based upon the amount of clinical income they generate and upon the discretion of their division chief. Notably, specialists employed in an academic setting and who perform clinical procedures, such as endoscopy, electroencephalography, vascular catheterizations, and echocardiography, can generate and share substantial additional income and bonuses. In contrast, pediatric nephrologists may be able to augment their income marginally from fee-for-service income alone. Thus, simply put, most pediatric nephrologists are not persuaded to enter their field by the prospect of a comfortable lifestyle or a lucrative salary.

Unlike private practitioners, most of those in academic medicine do not generally do their own patient billing and are not directly responsible for the clinic or office facilities, overhead costs, or salaries of the employees under their supervision. Having administrators handle these important but time-consuming business aspects, held a great appeal for me and was a major factor in my choosing an academic career. On the other hand, there are tradeoffs—nothing is free. Income generated from either clinical billing or from research grants must cover all salary and/or research laboratory costs and support other complicated arrangements related to medical-school affiliation. During the 1970's and 1980's salaries of academic physicians were predetermined, sometimes frozen for years, and generally much lower than those of private practitioners. This gross salary inequality is less prevalent in recent years. Also, the extent of clinical or research involvement and salary terms are typically negotiated with each physician prior to their hiring. Even physicians who are primarily designated as *physician scientists* or *researchers* are obligated to provide expert medical care, albeit on a limited time basis, and they are not exempt from teaching responsibilities. These physicians are expected to be productive in their research and are constantly under pressure to apply for outside grants to help support their salaries and laboratory expenses.

Prior to 1970, pediatric nephrologists embodied the *clinician, educator, scientist* triad, or "triple threat" model. The clinical demands associated with wide access to dialysis and transplantation after 1972 initially shifted this idealized balance such that there was less time for basic research. I am proud to say that nearly all pediatric nephrologists I have known over the years have placed the clinical needs of their patients above all other career objectives. Also, in my opinion, compared to other specialists employed in an academic setting, nephrologists have contributed disproportionately to the education of medical students and residents throughout the past five decades. However, as the U.S. nephrology workforce became sufficiently large to meet the clinical demand, an increasing number of graduates of nephrology fellowship programs have elected to pursue either predominantly clinical (patient care) or predominantly scientific (research) careers.

Personally, I modeled myself after the traditional "triple threat," and I believe that this is clearly apparent throughout this book. This challenge appealed to me a great deal because of my drive to overcome my modest beginnings in life and because of my strong competitive mentality. I had already demonstrated some talent as a triple threat during my residency and fellowship and had basked in the accolades of my superiors. This only reinforced my resolve to continue on the path of academic medicine. Although I never had formal instruction on teaching and researching, I thought that I could learn these on the job. I knew that this was a tall order, but my resolve was bolstered by my conviction that I did not have the desire, business mindset, or talents required to manage a private pediatric practice. However, implicit in academic medicine was the administrative responsibility of effectively managing a clinical division as well as a research laboratory. Despite dispensing these responsibilities for well over thirty years and accruing many new skills in the process, I must confess that I never developed a strong appetite for administrative duties. However, judging from the fact that I devote the bulk of this book to clinical medicine, I pursued this responsibility with much energy and passion. I derived great pride and joy from connecting with my patients and their families on a personal level and creating conditions conducive to optimal disease outcomes. The money would have been decisively better in private practice, particularly up front, yet because we lived modestly but comfortably, this did not influence my decision. I was quite idealistic and eager to remain at the forefront of medicine, testing new hypotheses and discovering mechanisms of disease that offered the prospect of novel therapies that could improve the health of children with complex medical disorders. Although such pursuits demanded a great deal of time and resulted in less money, I was thoroughly convinced that this lifestyle was more compatible with my general philosophies of medicine and life, as well as my overall idiosyncrasies. Fortunately, my wife was of the same mindset and she never wavered from supporting nearly all my professional endeavors.

The duties of academic physicians have gradually shifted over the years. Instead of the triple threat described above, each aspect is more clearly delineated now. On close review of my curriculum vitae one can easily infer that despite having a full clinical and teaching load, I managed to gain notable success in both basic and clinical research. Less obvious are the academic obligations that consume a large portion of time for all physicians in academic medicine, especially those in charge of their specialty. In my capacity as the director of pediatric nephrology, I had multiple other titles and responsibilities, such as medical director of pediatric renal transplantation, chairman of the medical library committee, director of the pediatric renal fellowship program, chairman of the Kidney Foundation Advisory Committee, and committee chairman of several ad hoc committees reviewing the qualifications for promotion of other colleagues. I was also responsible for the formal annual evaluations of all faculty and other personnel in my division. These reviews were then shared with the chairman of pediatrics and hospital administrators, and together, we determined salary changes and, if necessary, corrective actions. In addition, I served as mentor to my faculty and actively participated in multiple pediatric faculty committees and meetings. I conducted numerous interviews of pediatric residency program and renal fellowship applicants. I taught students at the medical school. As a member of the Human Rights Committee, I reviewed multiple of in-house research grants. I also met regularly with an increasing number of administrators to discuss clinic facilities, staffing issues, and billing. All these duties were fitted into a very busy clinical schedule, so twelve-to-fourteen-hour-long days were the norm rather the exception. However, as one can glean from reading this book, despite these chores, for me, the positives well outnumbered the negatives.

Promotion in academic rank
to full professor with tenure

<hr>

In the early 1980s, the medical staff at CHP was small and consisted of thirty-five seasoned, efficient, industrious, and highly respected physicians. In a true team spirit, they collaborated and supported each other to achieve the common goal of providing the best care possible to all children in Western Pennsylvania and West Virginia, despite minimal personnel and relatively few financial resources or community support. It seemed as if each member was a crucial part of the whole; collectively, we were stronger than we were individually. In this collegial environment, many physicians were able to fulfill their non-clinical requirements. This meant conducting research and publishing scientific articles, which eventually led to promotions and the accompanying and much-welcomed 10 percent salary raise. Consideration for promotion typically occurred every six years. Indeed, despite my exceptionally heavy clinical responsibilities, I was most privileged in 1984 to be promoted to associate professor in the tenured track. Getting promoted with tenure was among the highlights of my life, as my entire educational effort starting from grammar school on seemed to culminate in this singular achievement.

I recall being summoned in 1984 to meet with Dr. T. K. Oliver, the chief of pediatrics who recruited me first as a resident and then as director of pediatric nephrology, and who spearheaded my application for promotion. The reason for the meeting was undisclosed, causing some consternation on my part. Dr. Ellis Avner, who we had recruited to the pediatric nephrology staff four years earlier, joined us in Dr. Oliver's office. Dr. Oliver then made the glorious announcement and gave me his warm congratulations and a handshake. In his inimitable style, he interjected some trite humor, questioning the merit of my promotion, and then served champagne. At first, I was surprised and incredulous to learn of my promotion. The title "associate professor of pediatrics and nephrology with tenure, University of Pittsburgh, School of Medicine" was added to my previous title of director of pediatric nephrology at the Children's Hospital of Pittsburgh, which, while admittedly long, seemed to validate my work. At a similar celebration in 1990, I was informed that I was promoted to the rank of full professor with tenure. I was in total disbelief until several days later when I received the official letter from the president of the university confirming my promotion:

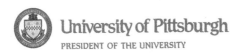

University of Pittsburgh

PRESIDENT OF THE UNIVERSITY

November 8, 1990

Dr. Demetrius Ellis
1015 Gilchrest Drive
Pittsburgh, Pennsylvania 15235

Dear Dr. Ellis:

It gives me great pleasure to approve the recommendation of Dean George Bernier, Senior Vice President Thomas Detre and Provost Donald M. Henderson that you be promoted to the rank of Professor in the Department of Pediatrics in the School of Medicine, effective January 1, 1991.

This promotion to the highest academic rank recognizes the promise implicit in the conferral of tenure has been fulfilled and expresses the University's confidence that your achievements are widely acknowledged by the community of scholars. We greatly appreciate your contributions to the University.

Warmest congratulations.

Sincerely,

Wesley W. Posvar
President

PITTSBURGH, PA 15260 (412) 624-4200

DEMETRI: A MODEL OF EFFICIENCY

STARTING MY CAREER as the chief and solo nephrologist at CHP, I was on call at all times of the day, particularly during the first three years. At all times, I was obligated to carry a primitive electronic pager with a single tone and have close access to a telephone, so I could call back the hospital operator and retrieve the message. Family vacation was out of the question during those early years, and I functioned strictly on survival mode. My only social outlet was soccer and tennis, which I squeezed into my schedule whenever possible. Recruitment of a second pediatric nephrologist was difficult at that time for several reasons—our pediatric program was not acclaimed, the workload was large and salaries relatively low, the number of nephrologists in the States was very small, the number of graduating nephrology trainees was miniscule, and Pittsburgh was not the attractive city that it is today. Thus, given my many duties and faced with a manpower shortage, I employed all shortcuts that would enable me to do my work as efficiently as possible, with the clear proviso that these shortcuts did not compromise patient care.

As part of my MO, starting early in my career, I made a concerted effort to educate physicians and nurses on the renal disorders of children under our mutual care. My intention was to motivate these physicians and nurses to review the renal condition pertinent to our patient. This was especially important for patients managed in the ICU by fellows and residents whose shifts changed daily. In contrast, ICU nurses tended to be assigned to the same patients for up to four consecutive days. Calling the ICU fellow for a clinical update on one of my patients consisted of a lengthy but predictable scenario: Paging him/her through the hospital operator and a prolonged telephone hold. Direct answers to my questions were rare. Rather, the fellow would reply that he/she would review the patient data and call me back. The fellow would then review the data, have a discussion with the nurse, discuss the case with his/her attending physician, and then call me back. By contrast, the assigned ICU nurse was nearly always at the bedside and could be reached by calling the patient room number directly. Most ICU nurses were very experienced and dedicated, and, having participated in the morning rounds, they were well-informed about the child's condition, laboratory information, and general daily management objectives. Therefore, they could supply the clinical information I needed with minimal prodding. In short, I was able to obtain an excellent and swift clinical update within minutes. I would then ask the nurse to inform the fellow of my assessment, recommendations, and suggestions with the option for the fellow or attending physician to call me back for any clarification. This approach greatly contributed to my efficiency and also led to more timely changes to the care of my patients. Because my approach did not intend to bypass the ICU fellow or deprive them of contributing their independent medical decisions, I made an extra effort to teach them whenever I encountered them in the ICU.

I highly respected the extraordinary dedication and professionalism of many nurses in the ICU, as well as those who worked closely with me in my renal division. Diane was exceptional in the ICU. However, MJ G personified pediatric nursing and took the cake when it came to providing total, comprehensive care, including home care and social services, long before the currently existing "wraparound services" that require a large team of health care providers to implement. Nancy W. and Carol R. were also the ultimate in competence, dedication, and professionalism.

One outstanding nurse, Patty H., was particularly involved in post-transplantation care. Perhaps because of my close interaction with her in caring for many critically ill children and my emphasis on how kidney dysfunction accounted for their clinical manifestations, Patty became intrigued and wished to acquire more than just a superficial knowledge about renal anatomy and function. She was genuinely eager to understand the nephrons, those magical, elegant, but functionally complex individual units that can affect the operation of each body cell and organ. Largely because of the obvious vigor and enthusiasm with which I explained to Patty and to the physicians at the ICU various aspects of nephron function, she referred to me as the "Nephron Man." I must have loved this appellation because soon after she coined this nickname, I wrote a rap song by the same title, shown below.

"NEPHRON MAN"
by Demetrius Ellis, M.D., alias Metanephros
(Marching theme song of the pediatric nephrologist)

Life is not always fair
Nephron Man do not despair
Let your full patient commitment
Be the road to high achievement

Hematuria? Hypercalciuria?
Hyperuricosuria?
Eyes swollen from proteinuria?
Find the diagnosis as quickly as you can

Growth failure and uremia?
Bone disease and anemia?
Nephrolithiasis, masquerading as nephritis
Will not escape careful urinalysis
There are no challenges for Nephron Man

It feels good to get filtration
After renal transplantation
Get rid of mechanical purification
Grow tall with steroid-free immunosuppression

Keep your eyes on the horizon
I say get down with the program
Bring on prednisone and Cytoxan
ACE inhibitors and losartan

Keep the emphasis on prevention
Hypertension regulation
Put a stop to renal-injury progression

Ellis to the table brings
Experience and common sense,
Minnesota Vats on grants
Gets along with research rats,
Moritz can fix electrolytes like no one can
Or, he can help you get to the promised land

Life is not always fair
Nephron Man do not despair
Let your full patient commitment
Be the road to high achievement

I went to see nephrology when I was just a lad,
And they told me the name of the condition I had.
Protein showed up in my urine when I had to go,
They took a look and told me that they definitely know—it's

Membranoproliferative glomerulonephritis
Elevated blood pressure that's not caused by bursitis
Your kidney biopsy and surely urinalysis still spell:
Membranoproliferative glomerulonephritis.

(Notes: Metanephros represents the more advanced stage
of embryonic development of the kidney. Dr. Vats- not
"Minnesota fats"-trained at the University of Minnesota and
is primarily a basic researcher. Dr. Moritz is a devout orthodox Jew and did clinical research in electrolytes.)

Patty H enrolled in night classes and eventually became an invaluable physician assistant embedded at the liver and small bowel transplant service at CHP. She also received a Ph.D. in nursing.

Introduction to patient anecdotes and lessons learned

———— ∽ ————

CHP: A clinical bonanza and an emotional rollercoaster

Although I could use the word *journey* to describe my career path, I think that *adventure* is a more apt term. Unlike a journey, which one can plan from the start, *adventure* implies an uncharted voyage without a specific destination and with many unexpected turns. It also implies that one may be exposed to potential dangers as well as have the prospect of making amazing discoveries. I experienced surprises and challenges at every turn, and this voyage consumed every ounce of my energy. Inevitably, it also elicited a menagerie of emotions.

Because acute or severe illness or trauma triggers many emotions or feelings that can directly or indirectly influence the outcome of these conditions, I have opted to briefly discuss this important aspect of health and healing. Unlike other members of the animal kingdom, humans are capable of expressing numerous emotions—each having a range of intensity—that can profoundly affect our behavior and, thusly, impact our survival. These emotions may erupt instantly and be conveyed through often complex yet unequivocal, readily recognizable facial expressions and distinct language, as well as predictable physiological alterations. For instance, anger and fear may be triggered by many real or perceived circumstances and manifest as distinct facial and body gestures, loud, vulgar and offensive language, increased heart and breathing rates, the proverbial visceral effect or "knot in the stomach," and flight response, all of which occur automatically and are sub-served by the release of adrenaline and cortisol by the adrenal glands. The portions of the brain called amygdala and hypothalamus may have a central role in perceiving and initiating these neurophysiologic responses through elaboration of regulatory proteins such as stathmin, and hormones including oxytocin and CRH. Furthermore, the intensity of the response may vary among individuals and may also be disproportionate to the triggering event. While such responses may project strength and resolve as to help protect one against an adversary or perceived threat, they may also provoke rather than discourage a fight with another individual. Moreover, the presence of a serious or potentially life-threatening illness can disrupt or interfere with our adaptive responses and impair our ability to manage our negative emotions. Clearly, excessive stress, anxiety, and depression sap away energy needed for body repair.

Although emotions are triggered without forethought, at a subconscious level, it is possible to raise awareness of a particular emotion and utilize tools that enable one to modify responses, thereby leading to healthier and more socially acceptable behavior. Tipping the balance from anger, apposition, apathy, hopelessness, anxiety, and grief toward more positive emotional responses, such as acceptance, courage, determination, and perseverance, is of vital importance- it helps channel our emotional and physical energy in a beneficial, rather than harmful, direction and thus help us overcome a serious illness or injury. Positive emotional responses may also enhance our compliance with medications, diet, and other lifestyle measures that indirectly contribute to healing and our will to survive. Ultimately, an appropriate balance of our emotions is fundamental to achieving joy and fulfillment in our lives.

Like other pediatricians, I have observed that even infants can express deep, complex emotions in response to social and environmental cues. Personally, I had the privilege of experiencing many intense emotions directly emanating from the circumstances of my patients as well as other joyous or stressful events related to my academic career. These feelings are evident in the anecdotes that follow. Note that even though many of these interactions took place years ago, the memories remain vivid and completely validate my decision to become a doctor in the first place; they also serve as affirmation of the ideals and passion associated with this noble profession. I believe that all readers will readily identify with the characters of the stories.

While these stories depict a variety of situations that inspire a range of emotions, I believe that they all convey a common, simple, yet enduring and important message: taking a genuine interest in the individual and not just focusing on his/her disease, empowers physicians to become more effective healers and brings fulfillment, contentment and joy to their lives. This and other lessons learned from my patient interactions culminate in a well-defined set of core principles listed in p. 209, my *Advice to my residents and fellows: Strive to be the best!* Several of these tenets are not new and are implicit or complementary to the precepts in the *Hippocratic Oath* (see p. 208). One may even say that they represent a "back to the future for medicine" direction. On the aggregate, however, I am convinced that they constitute the essence of contemporary medicine. In my humble opinion, these principles represent a road map for strengthening the trust and respect between physicians and patients that has eroded in recent decades, thereby enhancing our professional satisfaction. Thus, refocusing on these principles together with embracing scientific progress and reforms in health care policy as to promote, preserve and invigorate the unique holistic doctor-patient relationship, are very likely to benefit physicians and their patients as well (see p. 222, *The changing face of the medical profession).* Thus, health care recipients may also choose to obtain care from physicians who embody these principles.

While reading these anecdotes, I urge you to be mindful of the fact that, prior to 1990, health care delivery was less effective than today because of limited ancillary support resources and because several transformative technological and scientific advances had not yet materialized.

MUSICAL TEETH

Because a minimal amount of kidney-related lingo is essential to more fully appreciate this and other anecdotes throughout this book, please indulge me as I begin with a brief introduction on kidney function.

The kidneys are nearly identical twins, with identical function. Two are more fun than one, and, well, God, in His infinite wisdom, gave us two of these vital organs, so we can survive in case one of them was injured or failed. Thus, I will refer to the "kidneys" or "kidney" interchangeably. I am entirely convinced that the kidney is a charismatic, high-functioning, low profile, industrious, assertive, and no-nonsense organ. However, do not interpret this to mean that the kidney does not like to party. In fact, few, if any, organs are as interconnected, engaging, or as sociable as the kidney. The kidney filters the blood and gets rid of excessive fluid, metabolic and digestive byproducts, or ingested toxic chemicals. By doing this in a very meticulous manner, it maintains precise control of the chemical composition of the fluid that surrounds and enables each body cell to perform optimally. These functions are performed by about one million *nephrons* within each kidney, together with the participation of and in response to multiple hormones produced by the kidneys endocrinology cousins, including the pituitary, parathyroid, and adrenal glands.

However, from an evolutionary perspective, the most important function of the kidney is long-term blood pressure regulation through the development of elaborate but elegant and very clever mechanisms for conserving body fluids and regulating electrolytes. This vital function is mainly responsible for enabling our amphibian predecessors to venture beyond their primordial, water-dependent environment and survive on land. In fact, the preeminent twentieth-century physiologist

Homer W. Smith, in his book titled *From Fish to Philosopher*, makes a persuasive scientific argument that credits the development of the kidney with the evolution of early man and his subsequent attainment of higher-order thinking and creativity. As you can surely surmise, I am unable to restrain myself from extolling the kidney and its many virtues; indeed, I am the biggest fan of this marvelous organ.

It is easy to overlook other, perhaps less vital but important kidney functions. These less obvious physiologic functions tend to become manifest with debilitating symptoms or even death after prolonged or irreversible chronic renal injury that is not managed effectively. For instance, one of the many hormones produced by the kidney is an extremely active form of vitamin D (1,25 dihydroxy vitamin D3). This vitamin, coupled with the role of the kidney in handling calcium and phosphorus balance, is essential for maintaining bone health. Dysregulation of these processes results in compensatory secretion of parathyroid hormone that-in the course of progressive renal failure-may eventually become insufficient to contain this problem, leading to aberrant bone formation. This disorder is known as *secondary hyperparathyroidism*. In growing children, this is typically manifest by bowing and pain of the long bones of the lower extremities that is commonly referred to as *renal rickets*. This bone disorder, together with reduced secretion of another largely renal-derived hormone, called *erythropoietin*, limits red blood cell production in the bone marrow, causing anemia. Thus, severe anemia and associated generalized fatigue is ubiquitous among patients with advanced renal failure. The first patient anecdote exemplifies how groundbreaking pharmacologic advances have been highly effective in preventing or reversing these complications of chronic kidney failure, starting with *renal rickets*.

In 1977, at about noon on a Friday, I received a page from a dental resident. He informed me that the dental and general surgical teams had just admitted a five-year-old boy who had a large tumor on his lower jaw that appeared nearly transparent, or *radioluscent*, on X-rays. All the teeth of the lower jaw were said to be loose. The timing of this call related to the fact that routine preoperative blood testing had revealed an elevated serum creatinine (2.3 mg/dL), indicative of renal dysfunction. The surgery to remove a major part of the jaw and the suspected malignant osteosarcoma was scheduled only two hours later, so they needed me to evaluate him on a urgent basis.

The boy was short-statured for his age, wore black-framed eyeglasses with thick lenses, and had a markedly protruding jaw, or *prognathia*. His mother reported no prenatal complications and no medical history of unexplained fevers or other urinary symptoms to suggest a pre-existing disorder caused by urinary tract infections or urologic disorders. The boy had developed a habit of eating soft foods or soups because of the gradual loosening of his teeth and increasing gum tenderness over the prior six months; remarkably, he had not lost any of his teeth. He also seemed to be low on energy and complained of knee pain even after minor physical activity. He took no vitamins or medications of any kind. On physical examination, the child's lower jaw was slightly tender to touch, and the tumor was soft, rather than having a firm or bony consistency. No gingival inflammation was present, and the teeth were easily movable in all directions and seemed to be barely held in place mainly by the gum tissue. When I gently moved the teeth across on a horizontal plane, there was a soft musical cadence resembling the sound one domino makes when falling onto the next. No local cervical lymph node reaction or neck pain was noted. In addition, he had bowed legs and palpably widened distal femoral and tibial growth plates, or *metaphyses*, at the knees along with mild localized pain—all common signs and symptoms of active rickets.

On review of the X-rays, the tumor was large and radiolucent, and had largely replaced the bone structure of the jaw or mandible. Given the radiologic features, I suspected that this was a benign "brown tumor," so named because of the previously described slightly brown color of the tissue noted on gross pathologic inspection. The added findings of renal failure, rickets, and short stature suggested a primary chronic renal disorder. I obtained further X-rays of the distal clavicles, where brown tumors are generally more prevalent, and I found them on both clavicles. Given all the evidence, I was excited at the prospect of treating the child medically, without surgery. Thus, I persuaded the surgical team to obtain a simple biopsy of the tumor and postpone the planned major and disfiguring surgical procedure. In the meantime, I pursued further diagnostic tests and initiated appropriate medical and dietary management.

A subsequent renal ultrasound and voiding cystourethrography revealed small kidneys with abnormal contours and obstruction of urinary flow from the kidneys to the bladder. This was highly suggestive of a disorder descriptively known as *obstructive uropathy*. This condition is now classified under the spectrum of *congenital anomalies of the kidneys and urinary tract*, or CAKUT, and is a relatively common cause of chronic renal failure in children. The tumor biopsy confirmed the diagnosis of brown tumor, a condition resulting from intense osteoclastic activity and bone resorption. Secondary hyperparathyroidism was also confirmed by blood studies showing very high circulating levels of parathyroid hormone, together with low levels of vitamin D, and slightly reduced serum calcium but high serum phosphorus levels. I then discussed the pathophysiology of this condition with the parents, residents, and surgeons. I felt as though I had scored a hat trick and quickly gained much respect from my colleagues.

However, far more important than attaching a diagnosis is the successful management of a disorder. Three weeks after placing the child on a low-phosphorus diet, a calcium supplement, and a synthetic form of the biologically active 1,25 vitamin D3, that we had trialed at CHNMC in the prior two years, this boy's teeth became less mobile and the jaw tenderness resolved. Within three months, the tumor size had regressed, and the jaw was much less prominent. His teeth became anchored and he was now able to chew solid food. In addition, he was happier because he was able to play without experiencing knee pain. Over the past several decades, this and less egregious manifestations of skeletal demineralization have been largely controlled or prevented in nearly all patients with renal failure who are willing to comply with dietary, pharmacologic, and dialysis approaches.

Needless to say, the family was thrilled because their son had been "saved from surgery." The chief of pediatric dentistry, Dr. Mamoon Nazif, asked me to give a grand rounds lecture on this topic to his residents and students at the University of Pittsburgh, School of Dentistry. This was followed by an invitation to lecture on other dental disorders occurring in conjunction with advanced renal failure or uremia in children. This assignment encouraged me to expand my own knowledge on topics that I could not have imagined being in the purview of nephrology. For example, one interesting study showed that while excessive dental plaque was common among children with chronic renal failure, dental cavities were less prevalent compared to healthy children in the general population. This unanticipated benefit was attributed to increased blood urea nitrogen (BUN) level in the saliva of these "uremic" children, which was shown to retard the growth of the cavity-causing bacteria, lactobacillus.

The lecture on dental disorders in children with advanced renal failure became an annual event, and Dr. Nazif and I, as well as our wives and children, became close friends for life. This is just one of the many examples of how the kidney was my passport into learning as well as many lasting friendships throughout my career.

Eventually, the above child had a successful kidney transplant and is alive today. Because his unique clinical presentation and advanced secondary hyperparathyroidism with systemic osteoclast proliferation-driven skeletal demineralization and multilocular mandibular radiolucency compatible with brown tumor are of educational value, his picture and mandible X-rays are displayed in one of my publications (Atlas of Pediatric Physical Diagnosis. Davis H and Zitelli B (Eds), Gower Medical Publishing Ltd, New York, 2017, pp 455-479).

LET'S BALLET! (OR, THE BEAUTY AND THE GARDENIA MAN)

By five years of age, Laurel was a very accomplished ballet dancer. Of course, I did not know this when I first met her in the Emergency

Department of Children's Hospital of Pittsburgh in 1991. I was immediately struck not just by her marked skin pallor but also by her unusual, porcelain-doll-like facial features. (I was later informed that the parents achieved this effect by applying special skin creams.) She was truly a strikingly beautiful child. Apparently, Laurel developed bloody diarrhea within twenty-four hours of consuming a hamburger. Several days later, she developed severe anemia, extreme pallor and fatigue, and then stopped urinating. It quickly became apparent that she had hemolytic uremic syndrome (HUS) associated with an *E. coli* infection and that she had advanced acute renal failure. In fact, she rapidly achieved criteria for mechanical purification of her blood, or *dialysis*. Because of her gastrointestinal disorder and associated abdominal pain, I elected to employ *hemodialysis* instead of *peritoneal dialysis* (see p. 64). This required the insertion of plastic tubes in the large veins near the neck region that were connected to a dialyzer and a dialysis machine intermittently over the next five weeks (see p. 23). Laurel also developed pancreatitis and other complications of HUS resulting in a prolonged hospital stay.

During her hospital stay, I saw Laurel at least twice daily, and I became impressed with how attentive she was. She would look at me directly with an almost expressionless face and would not utter a word, nor would she smile. Her parents assured me that, in my absence, Laurel communicated with them in her typical fashion and had not indicated experiencing pain or other discomfort. In fact, Laurel's parents reassured me that she actually liked me and was not intimidated or fearful of me. In short, they had no explanation for her lack of interacting with me personally. In any case, I felt that it was important for me to explore and address Laurel's fears, concerns, and questions, as well as to make our daily interactions more pleasant. I reasoned that this would be good for Laurel's sake. I must confess, however, that I had selfish motives too. I felt defeated by the unnerving stare and silent treatment from such a young child. Thus, if I succeeded in breaking the ice, it would be a small but satisfying personal victory. However, an effective strategy for accomplishing this was not immediately apparent.

At about one week into Laurel's admission to CHP, I noticed a pair of small, pink ballet shoes by her pillow. These seemed more suitable for a large doll rather than for a child. However, on further inquiry, I discovered that Laurel had been enrolled in ballet classes since the age of two and that she had already auditioned successfully for several important ballet performances in Pittsburgh and elsewhere. This gave me an idea. I reasoned that no five-year-old child could resist a good laugh at the sight of a grown-up doing something foolish. So, one day about two weeks into her admission, after completing my morning bedside rounds and discussing Laurel's progress and the day's plans with my residents and with Laurel's parents, I decided to put my plan in motion. I stopped short of exiting the room, turned to Laurel, and with a serious yet casual manner, I said, "By the way, Laurel, last night I practiced a ballet routine that I saw on television, and I wonder if I could get your expert opinion on how to improve my technique." Laurel suddenly sat up straight, and I detected interest on her part, as if I had piqued her curiosity; she appeared intrigued. However, she did not say a word and, much like a seasoned poker player, refrained from showing a full facial expression. I then proceeded to take a ballet pose and made a very feeble attempt at a pirouette. I ran across the room with my arms extended and my legs apart, while my body turned 360 degrees in the air. At that point, Laurel, along with all others in the room, burst out in a loud laughter while I pretended to act embarrassed. Laurel then clearly and ably analyzed my pirouette, point by point, noting the multiple mistakes that I had made. Further, she promised that, the following day, she would demonstrate a proper pirouette. From that day on, I was able to engage Laurel in conversation, enabling her to show her emotions and vocalize her concerns. After two full months in the hospital, Laurel was sent home and gradually underwent full recovery.

While going through my stash of letters in preparation for this book, I came across the following song titled *Laurel's Tune* that her aunt had written while Laurel was in the hospital. For unknown reasons, the family did not share this with me until nearly seven years later. I believe this song captures the anguish and strength of faith of the extended family, as well as Laurel's courage and resilience while enduring this illness:

Laurel's Tune
(Chorus)
They've got a way to show they care,
A sort of essence in the air,
No matter what the time day or night,
You know they are always there.

At morning's light, it all seemed right
Like every day began.
A burger at a fast food place, and
Through the park she ran.
An hour on the see-saw, couple minutes on the swings.
Up and down the sliding board, and all the while
She sings.

Her little voice joins happily with birds who
Watch her play,
And passers-by wish they could be who Laura is
Today.

As darkness fell and day was done, night told a
Different tale.
This little girl so full of life,
Now fragile and so frail.

The stomach ached, her fever raged,
Such pain for one so young,
We thought this was our darkest night,
The worst was yet to come.

We raced to Children's Hospital,
While driving through our tears.
The doctors and the nurses there
Confirmed our darkest fears.

Her kidneys had now given up.
Her cheeks had lost their pallor.
But through it all the people there
Kept pace with faith and valor.
(Chorus)

Their thoughtfulness was always heard
In everything they'd say.
And never did we ever hear
"How are you going to pay?"

The days went by, then weeks and months
We never felt alone.
Their tender care and loving hearts
Made this our second home.

Time marches on. Now years have passed
Since Laura's second chance.
God's given her the gift and grace
And talent of the dance.

She runs and skips and sings her tunes.

11/30/99

Two years after Laurel's hospital discharge, I received a special invitation crafted by her, exclusively for me. It was written in calligraphy, on pink stationary with a pair of ballet slippers on the top and cut to the shape of a heart. The occasion was a special performance of *The Nutcracker* just prior to Christmas 1993, given by the Pittsburgh Ballet Theater for the enjoyment of the patients at CHP. I attended this performance, and it was indeed memorable; Laurel had the leading role, Clara. While doing her perfect pirouettes, she would flash a beautiful smile in my direction that served a clear reminder of my own weak but effective pirouette two years earlier.

Coincidentally with receiving *Laurel's Tune*, I received yet another beautifully crafted invitation from Laurel:

Dear Dr. Ellis

Pittsburgh Youth Ballet's Nutcracker is coming up, and Ashley — and I will be performing on December 4, 1998 at 7:30 p.m., at Bethel Park High School.

Ever since I was three years old I have dreamed of dancing the role of Clara on this special night, but it is also my 12th birthday.

It would mean a great deal to me if you could attend; not a day goes by that my family and I don't thank our lucky stars for you.

If you are able to attend, please let us know how many tickets you will need. Georgia can handle the delivery of the tickets to you.

Sincerely,

This was another truly exquisite performance that mesmerized and amazed the audience. Deservingly, Laurel received great applause and yells of "encore." Several years later, she graduated magna cum laude from Point Park University with a Bachelor of Arts in dance. She successfully auditioned and received roles at the New York Ballet Theater, Radio City's Christmas Spectacular, and the Pittsburgh Ballet, as well as elsewhere. Laurel is currently married and has been serving as a ballet instructor at the Pittsburgh Ballet Theater School, from which she had once graduated.

This encounter with Laurel reinforced my philosophies of not taking myself too seriously and the importance of getting to know children by taking a genuine interest in their activities and personal lives. This, in turn, translates into greater trust and a more effective management. Humor also tends to be a great antidote to depressing or stressful situations, such as any encounters with serious illness.

What is my dialysis machine doing on eBay?

One late evening in 1982, I received a call from an outlying town informing me that a male newborn with known marked dilation of the anatomical parts that collect and transmit urine from the kidneys to the bladder, *hydronephrosis*, had not voided during the first day of life. Otherwise, he was full term and appeared healthy, without any respiratory compromise. A postnatal ultrasound confirmed these prenatal findings and also revealed a reduced amount of renal tissue as well as an enlarged bladder with a thick muscular wall. These features in a male newborn are highly suggestive of the diagnosis of *posterior urethral valves*, in which a small flap of tissue in the urethra—the tube that connects the bladder to the outside opening of the penis—exerts a valve-like effect restricting the exit of urine. This is potentially a very serious disorder because severe obstruction starting at an early embryonic stage impairs normal renal development and reduces urine and amniotic fluid production thereby impeding lung development as well. Thus, I requested transport of the baby by ambulance for direct admission to CHP. He arrived around nine o'clock that evening, accompanied by his seventeen-year-old mother and a very dedicated social worker. The mother had no prior pregnancies and appeared socially interactive and healthy. The social worker was aware of the mother's previous arrests for prostitution. The infant's father was unknown, and the mother's only support was an older sister with a family of her own.

Our pediatric urologists at CHP concurred with my diagnosis of the baby and performed a relatively simple surgical procedure to sever the flap of tissue and optimize urine flow. In this newborn, the urine drainage and hydronephrosis improved, but urine output remained very low and kidney function improved only marginally. Thus, soon after surgery, I recommended starting *peritoneal dialysis* to purify the blood of toxic substances until a kidney transplant could be performed, one to two years later, when the infant was of sufficient size. Unlike hemodialysis that was described above, peritoneal dialysis is conducted via a Tenckhoff catheter that is surgically inserted inside the abdomen, tunneled under the skin, and exits near the belly button. A specially formulated fluid is then infused into the abdomen where it equilibrates with the extensive capillary system, thereby enabling removal of accumulated potentially harmful molecules from the bloodstream into that fluid, which is then drained and discarded. Typically, this cycle is repeated ten to fifteen times over a period of eight to ten hours overnight, and the entire process is automated, utilizing a peritoneal dialysis machine. This process is much less complex and safer to perform than hemodialysis, particularly in infants and young children, making it suitable for home use. Hence, we arranged for the mother to remain at the Ronald McDonald House near CHP and to begin training to perform peritoneal dialysis. She appeared invested in her baby's health and expressed an interest in being a kidney donor once her son reached an acceptable body size. She was bright and quickly became familiar with the medications, diet, and automated dialysis procedure. The maternal aunt was also trained to conduct dialysis and served as a backup. We then made the necessary arrangements for the customary home visit and delivery and installation of a newly designed dialysis machine, a new sink to handle dialysis fluid effluent, electrical outlets, and other accommodations—all expenses paid by Medicare.

About a month later, our dialysis nurse telephoned to inquire why the mother had not brought the baby to the clinic for the mandatory follow-up visit. She could not reach the mother and then called the baby's aunt. The aunt informed us that the mother, along with another co-worker had had an altercation with their pimp. As a result, the mother had left town a week earlier; her whereabouts were unknown. In the meantime, the child was staying with the aunt. The aunt guesstimated that the last dialysis session had taken place the day prior to the mother's departure. She said that, because the baby appeared well, and the mother was expected to return and resume dialysis soon, she did not feel the urgency to notify the dialysis staff. This prolonged period without dialysis was concerning from a medical standpoint, so we arranged for an immediate evaluation of the baby at a local emergency department. To our surprise and great relief, his physical examination was satisfactory, and blood chemistry tests did not reveal any serious derangements resulting from impaired kidney function. We then requested a report on the status of the dialysis machine. Upon searching the mom's apartment, the aunt was unable to locate it. We suspected that the mother may have sold it. When we browsed on eBay we found several dialysis machines for sale, including the one matching our patient's make and home address. Fortunately, it had not yet been sold, and after a more thorough search, it was found in the attic, in its original package. Apparently, the infant had regained sufficient renal function as to permit delay in restarting dialysis two months later.

Noah's Princess

One of my patients, a thirteen-year-old named Noah, had end-stage renal failure and needed dialysis and renal transplantation. He was one of twelve Amish siblings ranging in age from ten months to twenty years. He was always dressed in traditional Amish attire consisting of black trousers and a solid blue shirt. His shirt was held in place by straight pins, which is the custom for women's rather than men's dress according to Old Order Amish tradition. It took several minutes and great care to detach these pins, so I could properly examine Noah in the clinic. I assumed that this outfit was acceptable because, being a child, Noah would not be embarrassed by wearing such attire. Similarly, his mother was wearing multiple layers of blue-colored dress material held together by straight pins. (Once, I dreamed that I visited Noah at his home and saw thousands of straight pins of all sizes that were used to hold together the clothing of all fourteen members of the household, including the baby's clothes.)

Noah was always pleasant, had a great smile, and was well behaved and cooperative during my exams. However, there was one major problem; we had no verbal interaction. His mother assured me that he was a chatterbox at home, but no matter what I asked him, for over two years, I could never get him to utter a single word.

At one clinic visit, during my usual small-talk, one-way conversation with Noah and his attentive mother supplying the replies to my questions, I received a clue that I thought might help me break this gnawing silence. Specifically, I learned that his assigned task at the family farm was to take care of a Horse and several other smaller animals. At this point, I recalled the ploy I had used successfully with Laurel and thought, if I said something silly or unreal pertaining to horse care it may entice him to engage in conversation. So, at an opportune time during a subsequent clinic visit, I casually mentioned to Noah that I was thinking of getting a horse. There was one thing that kept me from going ahead with this decision: I just could not figure out what to do with all that manure.

His demeanor suddenly changed; he looked at me with a shine in his eyes, a glow to his face, and a smile that bespoke of his complete confidence in the answer. Yet, to my surprise, he still said nothing.

At the next clinic visit, Noah presented me with a hand drawing and an accompanying black-and-white picture of his pony (shown below). I commended him on his amazing drawing and asked what his pony's name was. With a smile and glimmer in his eyes, he answered, "Princess," and then proceeded to tell me all about his horse. In fact, because he was Princess's main caretaker, Noah had the privilege of naming her. He was never silent after that visit. I still recall this incident as the horse that broke Noah's silence.

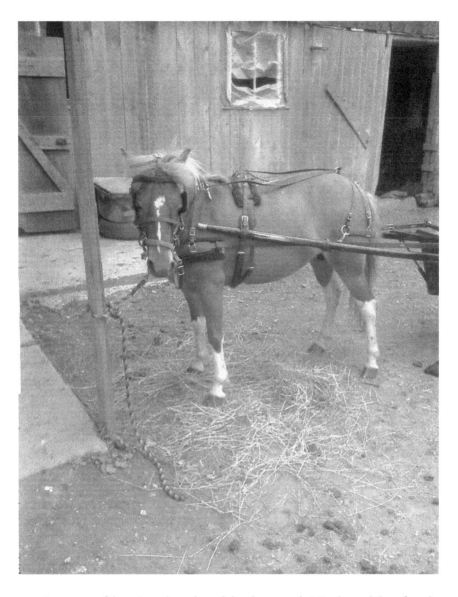

Because of his Amish cultural background, Noah and his family endured many more hardships than families facing comparable chronic medical conditions. His family was quite large, and although the older siblings helped take care of the younger ones, Noah's congenital renal disorder meant his care rested mainly with his mom. His father worked long hours, and therefore, he rarely accompanied his son to the renal clinic. Just arranging to come to clinic was a monumental task. They relied on the kindness of a non-Amish neighbor and friend who lived a couple miles away from them. This man remained in his car throughout the visit because he could not afford the parking fee. He shared a packed lunch with Noah and his mom. Our social service staff provided gas money, but the family was too proud to accept any additional financial assistance.

Even aspects of care that pose minimal hardship to mainstream society can be very troublesome to the Amish. For example, when the time came for Noah to start peritoneal dialysis, we were informed that the elders in their Amish community prohibited the use of electricity inside Noah's home. However, it was permissible for the peritoneal dialysis machine to be physically located and be used inside the house, so long as the electricity itself was not generated inside the home. Given these constraints we procured a gas-driven generator and installed it just outside of the home. Finally, after appropriate training at the dialysis unit of CHP, the mother proved very capable of conducting life-sustaining dialysis at his home. In fact, Noah's rate of infectious and other complications that typically occur in association with peritoneal dialysis was far lower than the norm.

Another important obstacle was securing payment for the expensive medical services related to advanced kidney failure, also known as end-stage renal disease. Because the Amish do not contribute to Social Security, they are not eligible for Medicare services that normally defray such expenses. Hence, for many Amish, the cost for dialysis and transplantation is typically incurred by their own community fund. Second, for religious reasons, the Amish circumvent organ donation from living donors but do approve of deceased donor renal transplantation. Because it is impossible to predict when such organs may become available and because of limited viability after harvesting from the donor, these organs must be transplanted expeditiously. Thus, once Noah's family opted for transplantation, it became essential to establish direct communication between the family, the dialysis and transplant nurse support staff, and the renal physicians. This presented yet another challenge, since the elders did not allow use of electricity or regular batteries inside the home. Eventually we solved this problem by procuring a solar-powered telephone, which was permissible by the community elders.

Despite the financial and emotional stress associated with facing a serious illness with an unpredictable outcome, both Noah and his mother appeared to cope well and, somewhat paradoxically, even seemed content and upbeat, at least outwardly. Their faith and trust in God was paramount, and perhaps enabled this Amish family to be accepting of the disease and at peace with themselves, regardless of the outcome. Noah eventually underwent a successful kidney transplant at fifteen years of age.

Notably, soon after Noah's transplant, I began my transition toward retirement, and due to my limited clinical schedule, I no longer had frequent interaction with my transplant patients, including Noah. However, when Noah was seventeen, my nurses informed me that he had assumed greater responsibilities at his family's farm, appeared healthy, pleasant and generally content during his routine transplant clinic visits at CHP, and often inquired about me. He was still a man of few words, which is reflected in his heart-felt letter to me upon my retirement (see p. 243).

Precious

Early in my career, I encountered a thirteen-year-old girl and her parents who lived in the Appalachian Mountains of West Virginia. She was referred to me for management of renal insufficiency associated with vesicoureteral reflux. In this relatively common congenital disorder that predominantly affects females, there is an anatomical impairment at the tubes that normally conduct urine from the kidneys strictly in a downward direction toward the bladder. This anomaly permits urine to go back up, or reflux, from the bladder in a retrograde direction. When reflux is severe and particularly when associated with recurrent urinary tract infections starting soon after birth, it can result in *reflux nephropathy* and severe kidney failure. Her father was a sharp, sprightly eighty-one-year-old while her mom was in her late forties. Both the father and the girl had striking West Virginian accents. Thus, I departed from my custom of interacting directly with my older patients and, to establish more clear rapport, directed my questions to the mom, whose speech was much easier for me to understand. The girl was attentive but fidgety and seemed to be very amused by my accent. After I asked her a question, she would turn to her mom and with her thick accent and a perplexed grin she said, "What did he say?" Mom would translate; then the girl would turn back to me and say something, to which I could only reply with a similarly perplexed smile. I would then turn to her mom and ask her to translate her daughter's words to me. This went on for a prolonged time during that initial visit.

As months and years passed, the girl and I figured out each other's accents sufficiently enough to communicate without needing an intermediary. When she was a senior in high school, she asked me to attend her graduation, and, as an incentive, she offered to let me ride Precious, her twelve-hundred-pound hog that had won first prize at the local animal fair.

My encounter with this girl and other families from West Virginia encouraged me to learn more words and expressions, some of which are common or unique to this community; a selected glossary is shown below:

Book read — educated
Peck — a whole lot of
Molasses — someone who moves way too slowly or like a turtle; not a syrup
Yunder — some measure of distance
Peperoni roll — something so good you can eat every day
Holler — a measure of distance; when you ask how far a place is, the reply may be, "It's a hoot and a holler."

Red up — means to tidy up, as in "tidy up your room"

Poke — a grocery bag

Buggy — store cart for your groceries

Go and see Miz Murphy — go to the outhouse

Got caught — to become pregnant

Hold your tater — be patient

THE AMAZING SISTERS
JOY AND CHERYL, AND THEIR PARENTS

During my initial encounter with them in 1981, I immediately realized that Joy and Cheryl, aged five and seven, were exceptional girls. Their parents were equally amazing; they were the embodiment of unconditional love and devotion. Their father was a well-educated forester, and the mother was a teacher. They had just relocated from the Philadelphia area to the mountains of West Virginia where the father was newly assigned and, hence, transferred their nephrology care to me at CHP. Both girls were markedly short, with striking facial and head derangements or *dysmorphism*. They had long head with diminished width known as *dolichocephaly*; sparse hair, abnormal nails, and pointed, peg-shaped teeth because of ectodermal dysplasia; small chest and slightly impaired lung function; hip and other skeletal problems; and small mal-developed kidneys and associated advanced renal failure. This constellation of features was consistent with the clinical diagnosis of Jeune syndrome. In this rare disorder each unaffected parent contributes a single copy of one of several implicated mutated genes. Unfortunately, genetic testing was not reliable at that time. Apparently, after Cheryl's diagnosis, the parents were led to believe that the chances of having another affected child was small. To their great dismay, however, Joy's distinctive physical features, or phenotype, were even more exaggerated than in Cheryl.

Both children were managed by peritoneal dialysis that their parents performed in an exemplary fashion. Both were schooled at home and excelled in reading, math, and science. Despite travelling two and a half hours each way every two months to my clinic, they were always pleasant, alert, energetic, and eager to see me. When I asked the girls, "Tell me everything that is new and exciting in your life," I was never disappointed to learn of their educational progress and family adventures.

After several clinic visits, I developed a close friendship with the family, and I devised a game that I thought would make the children's visits with me more bearable. I would ask each of them a trivia question, and if they answered correctly, I would give them a dollar. After several clinic visits without a single wrong answer, I decided I needed more challenging questions. Hence, prior to their subsequent visit, I sought my wife's help. She taught third grade at that time. Of course, she provided me both the questions and the answers, and the next morning, I walked into the tiny clinic room where only Cheryl was present. When I asked why Joy had not come, I heard a squeal from under the examining table. There, I found Joy crouched in a small, empty box that had contained printer paper. She jumped out and with a big smile she hugged me.

I then partially closed my eyelids, looked towards them sideways, and with a very serious professorial face I proceeded to ask my question being confident that, this time, I would stump them: "In the story of *The Wonderful Wizard of Oz*, what is the name of Dorothy's dog?"

Simultaneously, they answered, "Which of their dogs?" My face must have turned visibly red; I only knew of Toto. I was embarrassed to learn there were two dogs; I was also poorer by losing yet another two dollars.

On another clinic visit in September 1983, then seven-year-old Joy informed me that, during the preceding summer, she had accompanied her father to work and had become very interested in *entomology*. With minimal coxing, she proceeded to rattle off the scientific names, including genus and species, of numerous insects that she could describe in very impressive detail. She referred to the monarch butterfly as *Danaus plexippus*, while *Melanoplus differentialis* referred to the differential grasshopper, a species of grasshopper found in the United States.

By living in a nurturing, loving environment, both girls had been shielded against bullying and ridicule at school and escaped the stares of unknowing strangers. Consequently, they had abundant self-esteem, good work ethics, and great educational foundations, all of which served them well when they eventually attended college. They both underwent successful living donor kidney transplantation, Cheryl from her mom in 1984 and Joy from her dad in 1986. Both kidneys functioned very well. On last contact, Cheryl had married a young man who was 6' 4", but, clearly, it was the 4' 6" Cheryl who oversaw that household. I lost touch with Joy after she completed college but, assuming continued good health, I am certain she has also succeeded in her endeavors.

HALLOWEEN AT CHP

One of my all-time favorite fiascoes occurred during a Halloween party at CHP about twenty years ago. This event was organized by members of the "Play Therapy" team who assisted sick children and their families in making Halloween costumes, followed by the typical trick-or-treating and costume contest. Such events helped entertain and maintain a semblance of normal life during hospital stays. Although not formally stated, it was implied that adults and especially hospital personnel were excluded from participation, and that the event was for the benefit of the children. Despite this understanding, one of my residents—who is currently a renowned virologist—together with another resident and me decided to crash the party. Thus, we dressed up as kidneys, ureters, and bladder (see photo below). Both residents hung cardboard around their necks cut and painted to resemble kidneys, and each had a plastic tube connecting them to me—I was dressed as the bladder. A small pumpkin borrowed from the Halloween-decorated children's playroom hung between my legs and represented the bladder. We attracted a lot of attention as we paraded side by side around the hospital hallways, and later, we unashamedly received an award for *original costume design*.

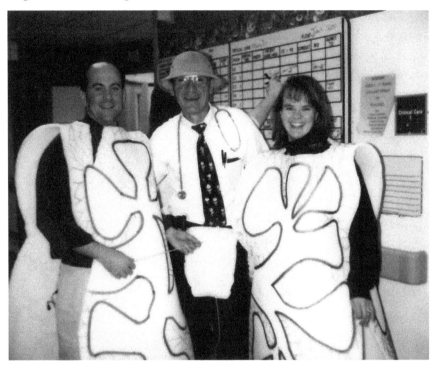

MORE HUMOR

Another time, I was making rounds with medical students and residents. On our way out of a patient's room, my eleven-year-old patient asked if he could ask me a personal question. Although I had no idea what he would ask and suspected that it could lead to an awkward situation, I guardedly agreed. He then said, "I noticed that you and the other nephrologists in your group all have foreign accents. I was thinking of becoming a pediatric nephrologist, but I want to ask you: Do you have to be a foreigner to be a nephrologist?" We all found this very amusing. I reassured him that he could proceed with his dream without such concerns.

On yet another occasion, my fellows, residents, students and I were at the bedside of a tall and husky sixteen-year-old male who was in good health but had elevated blood pressure. He also had attention-deficit-hyperactivity disorder (ADHD) and anger management issues that landed him in the George Junior Republic detention facility. One of my residents was reciting the medical history while I was performing my customary physical exam and noticed a large draining sinus, or hole, in his lower mid-back region above his anal opening. I asked the youngster if he was aware of this hole near his anus, to which he replied, "What?" I repeated the question. This time, he frowned at me and with an even more perplexed look on his face, he gave me the same reply. I asked him if he had noticed any drainage from near his ass, to which he emphatically replied, "No". The residents broke out in laughter, to the point of tearing as my conversation proceeded with questions about his testes and other parts of his anatomy using somewhat crude or vulgar language. This illustrates the importance of using vocabulary that is suitable for the cultural and educational level of the child and his/her family in communicating medical information.

FEAR

On one occasion in 1981, during my fourth year as a staff pediatric nephrologist, I was involved in the care of a sixteen-year-old boy, T. J., who needed urgent dialysis because of a life-threatening ingestion of antifreeze. Earlier that day, the boy's father had gifted him a brand-new car for his sixteenth birthday. In the early afternoon of the same day, the boy was driving at a high rate of speed with three of his friends, all of whom sustained superficial injuries when he crashed the car. When the police brought T.J. home, he and his father had a vociferous fight. The father threatened to confiscate the car keys and not repair it. His son replied that if his father went through with these threats he "had no reason to live anymore."

At about seven thirty that evening, T.J. was found sited on the floor of the garage next to the wrecked car; he was mentally confused and had incoherent speech. An empty container of antifreeze was open and partially spilled next to him. He was brought to the West Penn

Hospital Emergency Department, and three hours later, at midnight, he was transferred to my care at CHP. By that time, he had already progressed into a coma and had deep and slow respirations. Laboratory studies revealed a high blood ethylene glycol level and associated elevated osmolar gap of forty-five-conditions that favored development of brain swelling. Despite receiving large infusions of intravenous crystalloid and bicarbonate fluid for hydration, urine output was markedly reduced. Other findings included low blood calcium levels, large numbers of calcium oxalate crystals on urinalysis, increased blood acidity, and laboratory evidence of impending acute kidney failure. These studies together with the clinical features and circumstantial evidence were highly consistent with severe ethylene glycol -antifreeze- poisoning. The recommended treatment for this level of severity within a relatively brief time since the ingestion was ethyl alcohol (ethanol, as familiarly present in alcoholic beverages) combined with hemodialysis. Ethanol can be administered intravenously, as a drug, or in the form found in alcoholic beverages (hard liquors) delivered directly into the stomach via a plastic tube inserted via the nose. This treatment strategy, albeit strange on the surface, is scientifically sound. It is based on the fact that ethylene glycol is metabolized in the liver by the action of the enzyme alcohol dehydrogenase, thereby producing several toxic molecules, including glycolic and glyoxylic acids. Both of these acids are then converted to oxalate, which is insoluble and causes renal failure by precipitating in the kidney as calcium oxalate. This leads to decreased filtration of the blood by the kidneys (decreased GFR), resulting in decreased elimination of these toxic compounds, as well as production of formic acid, which can lead to blindness. Ethanol is also metabolized by the exact same enzyme, but it preferentially binds with it as to minimize the metabolism of ethylene glycol. Simultaneously, purification of the blood by mechanical means, or hemodialysis, enhances removal of any additional nonmetabolized ethylene glycol entering from the gastrointestinal tract into the circulation, and thus attenuates further toxicity. The key objective of management is to avoid lasting injury to the brain, retina, and kidneys and enable recovery of liver toxicity. (Notably, after 1997, fomepizole has been used to block alcohol dehydrogenase more effectively and thereby limit the neurologic and other toxic effects attributed to ethanol when this agent is employed as the antidote.)

While T. J. was being transferred to CHP ICU, I had already arranged to place a catheter in the subclavian vein as to start hemodialysis on an urgent basis and administer ethanol by vein. In the process of dialyzing T. J., I depleted all the intravenously approved ethanol supply of CHP and adjoining Presbyterian University Hospital pharmacies. However, within a couple of hours, T. J.'s blood ethanol levels began to fall, and he still had a high blood ethylene glycol level and elevated osmolar gap. At that time, we were employing hemodialysis fluid obtained by a reverse osmosis water generation system. This fluid was reconstituted with a special electrolyte mixture stored in an ordinary open-top metal tub next to T. J.'s bed in the ICU. This tub looked more suitable for bathing a small child than for dialysis use. However primitive by today's standards, this tub's design permitted easy access for adding ethanol directly into the water bath. I then located and used up two bottles of ordinary whiskey that I slowly mixed in the dialysis water bath.

TJ's father was obviously anxious and emotionally stressed by his son's serious medical condition. In addition, he appeared confused and could not comprehend my simplified explanation of the scientific basis of the treatment plan. He seemed especially skeptical of the concept that keeping his son drunk was of benefit in overcoming the antifreeze poisoning.

Meanwhile, ethylene glycol levels begun to decline at a good rate, and other blood parameters improved as well. Blood pressure and other vital signs remained stable, urine output picked up, and T. J. showed an improvement in his "coma score," all signs suggesting reversal of the overall toxicity. Thus, after eight continuous hours, I discontinued the dialysis.

Throughout that night, T. J.'s father took what seemed copious notes about my every move and of the conversations that I exchanged with the ICU personnel in connection with T. J.'s care. He was overtly agitated, pacing constantly while giving me an occasional angry glance. At one point, while holding what seemed to be the handle of a revolver on the right side of his undershirt, he came close to my face and in an angry tone said, "I will hold you responsible if anything goes wrong with my son."

I took this remark seriously and in the early morning, I reported the incident to our hospital security personnel. After a few telephone calls, the police discovered that the father had connections to the mob. Luckily, T. J. gradually improved. However, early during his recovery, he was combative and irrational. For about a week, he loudly showered the nurses and other caretakers who entered his room with four-letter words and other profanities. Such behavior is not unusual in individuals with liver dysfunction secondary to alcoholic cirrhosis or acute liver failure related to ethylene glycol intoxication. When T.J. visited me in my clinic two months later, he hugged me and, with genuine tears in his eyes, said, "Thank you for saving my life." He admitted that what he had done was stupid and vowed to make better decisions in the future. Unfortunately, many intentional overdoses are fatal and do not resolve any problems, no matter how significant these may seem at the time.

ELATION

While I experienced many joyous events during my career, nothing can compare with the two consecutive years of 100% graft and patient survival in some forty-five children transplanted at CHP in the early nineties. The team effort and emotional chemistry between our nephrology, ICU, nursing and surgical staff, including Ron and Velma from transplantation surgery, was so energizing and emotionally satisfying. For me, that feeling of elation during those two "perfect seasons" surpassed any personal joy I experienced as an athletic overachiever. Shortly after arrival from the OR to the ICU, I would evaluate and stabilize the child and then formulate a personalized treatment plan to be implemented in conjunction with our ICU staff. I would then meet with the anxious families and give them the good news they had so eagerly anticipated. One could tell that a huge weight had been lifted. The prospect that their children could now embark on new lives, unencumbered by the burden of dialysis and frequent hospital visits, as well as lifting of dietary and activity restrictions, was a dream come true. Indeed, their children would be able to take their first steps toward becoming successful and confident citizens, and the entire family could finally assume a semblance of a more predictable routine and lifestyle. My close involvement with the children and their families through the difficult transition of dialysis and transplantation gave me a greater appreciation of the sacrifices families made and especially of the courage of the parents, who were often the kidney donors. I was not just aware but also envious of the courage and resilience of the children who persevered and overcame multiple surgeries and serious complications.

Bobby's sad predicament—
A paradigm of raw courage and resolve

If I am permitted to boast, throughout my career, I had considerable success in managing many medical disorders and thus helped to enrich the development and futures of the children entrusted to my care. However, the circumstances of the children with poor outcomes remain much more vivid and haunting—they have left large, indelible scars deep in my mind. It is as if I can still see before me Danny and Susan and Karen, and Nilsy, and Mamas, especially as I grow older and have less daily contact with patients to occupy the active or "running" portion of my memory. These exceptional individuals and their families share many qualities and social threads. Bobby's story is particularly poignant and serves as a constant reminder that my chosen profession is far from being perfect or glamorous; there is blood, sweat, and tears to go around. This realization engenders helplessness and humility, and the need to seek guidance from a higher, divine being.

Bobby was a tall, assertive, and determined fifteen-year-old, who excelled in four sports. During the three months before I first met him in the late 1970s, he developed fatigue, mild shortness of breath, decreased appetite, and weight loss. These features led to routine laboratory tests, including a urinalysis that revealed the presence of an underlying renal disorder. In fact, he had advanced kidney failure evident by a serum creatinine of 4.0—the same as his GPA. The nasal septum, or membrane that separates the nostrils, had a hole in it, and the bridge of his nose was depressed. This constellation of findings suggested the diagnosis of Wegener's granulomatosis, a serious and progressive condition caused by inflammation of the blood vessels, or *vasculitis*, primarily involving the kidneys and lungs. Although this disorder is quite rare in children, his renal biopsy was consistent with this condition; it also revealed extensive scarring, reflecting severe, irreversible injury that portended poor response to any treatment intervention. As predicted, he only had marginal and transient benefit from intravenous infusion of Cytoxan, a chemotherapeutic agent that was the treatment of choice available at that time. He subsequently went on to have two episodes of lung, or pulmonary, hemorrhage that caused progressive difficulty with breathing.

Within two months, Bobby's condition reached a critical point; he lacked the energy to breathe or speak. He became dependent on the C-PAP apparatus-(continuous positive airway pressure)-that assisted with breathing, and he communicated principally through the aid of a board with alphabet letters that he used to spell out words and a few key phrases to which he could simply point. Yet Bobby did not appear deterred or discouraged by his progressive symptoms. He continued to put full effort into respiratory and physical therapy, took all his medications without fussing, and struggled but maintained his oral as well as supplemental nutrition given by a nasogastric tube. However, it became clear to all caretakers and to Bobby's parents that, to survive, he urgently needed a lung transplant, which was not offered because effective immunosuppression was not available at that time and this treatment modality carried a nearly 100% fatality. Without the prospect of lung transplantation, I could not recommend renal transplantation. Dialysis would also serve as a temporary measure, and because of the need for anticoagulation associated with this procedure, his preexisting risk of pulmonary (lung) hemorrhage would be exacerbated, hence, hastening his demise. In short, Bobby was facing the ultimate "catch-22".

At this impasse, we convened a multidisciplinary care conference that included all caretakers, a bioethicist, and Bobby's parents and adult siblings. First, Bobby's medical condition was reviewed in detail. The ICU staff felt that he had reached the point that intubation and ventilator support was imminent. In addition, he would require nutritional delivery via a gastric tube surgically inserted directly into the stomach, along with other life-sustaining measures. With such a dismal outlook, everyone, including Bobby's family, concluded that it was unethical to subject him to such invasive procedures. Because Bobby's cognitive function remained exceptional, it was also concluded that we should explore his personal understanding of his outlook and determine how far he wanted us to proceed. Given my close relationship to Bobby over the prior six months, it was suggested that I be the one to broach these issues with him. This was not a bridge I had crossed before. However, I accepted this task.

First, as sensitively and empathetically as I could, I summarized Bobby's medical condition and presented the upcoming issues facing him. When I finished, I asked him how he wished us to proceed. He then calmly and resolutely took his alphabet pad and spelled, "What is the alternative?" His answer was brief, but his facial expression spoke volumes; it said, "what choice do I have? Of course, I would do whatever is needed to stay alive". With these few words, he expressed so much and reinforced what I had suspected all along—the idea of giving up on a challenge was foreign to him and never entered his mind. "You have the choice of not accepting invasive procedures," I replied.

It seemed like, at that particular moment, Bobby had an epiphany—he finally realized that he would not survive. In an instant, all hope visibly vanished from his face. He suddenly became angry and combative, and despite his weakened condition, he began to pull out his nasogastric tube and intravenous lines. He then removed his C-PAP connections. This interruption together with his sudden burst of energy and oxygen consumption caused his blood oxygen level to fall precipitously and his lips to turn blue. We increased the oxygen that was now administered by face mask and gave him a small dose of sedation, enough to calm him down but not to compromise his spontaneous respirations. This produced the desired effect; however, his oxygen saturation gradually diminished over the next hour and he expired. In their typical quiet dignity, his loving family grieved by his side. The strength of character etched on the face of their brave and wonderful son and brother was unrivaled. Though Bobby's raw courage in the face of death was inspiring, his passing marked one of the darkest periods of my career.

I had hoped never to face such emotionally trying experience ever again. However, two decades later, another promising young man named Mamas had an equally devastating death, this time related to an accidental bleed in his chest following placement of a dialysis catheter. I admired these teenagers very much and often wonder where they would be today and what they would have achieved for themselves and for society if they'd had the opportunities to fulfill their potential.

These and other children with poor outcomes taught me what true courage is and the importance of keeping hope alive. In concert with the application of proven scientific interventions, I believe that hope is a real yet intangible trait that contributes to self-healing. Bobby's case forced me to reconsider how much hope I should convey to my patients, especially to teenagers who are capable of fully understanding their medical condition and prognosis. In Bobby's case, I felt that by giving him the impression that I was optimistic until the very end, I had lied or misrepresented his outlook—that I betrayed him in the end. This was a painful conclusion and indeed influenced my subsequent approach with families facing similar incurable conditions.

However, as I gained greater perspective, I developed a better appreciation of the importance of hope in healing. I also came to realize that I could not permit my grief and depression to persist and deter my efforts to help other children; I owed it to Bobby and Mamas, among others, to amass the strength and medical skills that would allow me to offer the prospect of hope and a better tomorrow to other children. Indeed, given the advances in medicine and transplantation, individuals with Wegener's granulomatosis currently have a much better outlook.

Several other families had maintained communication with me for many years after I had first interacted with them or even after the death of their child. During my major professional crisis (see p. 193), Bobby's mother submitted a letter to a newspaper strongly supporting my stance on the part of my patients. Her words reflected the strong bond that had formed between us several years earlier and were most welcomed and uplifting. I believe that my perspective on hope was of great value to these families.

Susan's social and medical nightmare

Susan is among the children I most admired. She was a ten-year-old known to me since infancy. Just like the girl described earlier in "*Precious*," Susan had reflux nephropathy but much more advanced chronic renal failure together with marked blood pressure elevation. She had yet another admission to CHP to control an acute exacerbation in high blood pressure that resulted in severe headaches and visual impairment, medically referred to as *malignant hypertension*. The blood pressure and symptoms responded well to a powerful medication given continuously by vein in the ICU and she was quickly transitioned to her oral medications and low-sodium diet. This was a recurrent scenario, raising suspicion of lack of adherence with these same measures at home.

Two days later, Susan felt well enough to participate in a play therapy session. Apparently, the play therapist was so astonished at what Susan had drawn that she felt compelled to page me to come down and see it for myself. It was a cartoon likeness of me examining a child, complete with a medical coat, eyeglasses, and stethoscope. While I routinely and intentionally invited my patients to have fun at my expense, this was the first time that one of them had portrayed me in a cartoon. A balloon held by the child read "In case of emergency, first call Dr. Ellis, then my priest and then my mother." Boy, did Susan have her priorities messed-up!

Among nearly all disadvantaged children that I cared for during my many years of practice, Susan best exemplifies the detrimental influence of the socioeconomic status on chronic disease outcome. In fact, her socioeconomic predicament may have been primarily responsible for her eventual demise. Susan's parents had been separated for about three years. Her father was abusing alcohol and drugs and had abandoned the family; reportedly, he was homeless in Baltimore. Susan, her eight-year-old brother, her mother, and her grandmother lived together in her maternal grandmother's home. Both adults were poor and uneducated. Susan's mother was a low-key, pleasant woman who labored to make ends meet. She was never bitter or express anger about her plight. She simply responded to life's blows by rolling with the punches. She clearly loved her children very much and worked as a nurse's aide at a state-run home for senior citizens. She took two buses to go to work and had no time for a social life.

When Susan was eleven years old, it became apparent that she needed dialysis and/or renal transplantation. Her mother was not a suitable match, and, after much effort and resourcefulness, our social service worker managed to locate Susan's father, who consented to be evaluated as a prospective donor. Arrangements were made for his transportation to Pittsburgh and for lodging at the Ronald McDonald House. I first met up with him late one evening at the ward where Susan had been admitted. It was clear from his appearance and odor that he was living on the street, and soon after our introduction, he asked me for dinner money. I gave him some of my pocket money, and that was the last time I saw him. Apparently, he remained in town for a couple more days and had preliminary blood studies. He then had second thoughts and left town without completing his evaluation or leaving behind any contact information.

Several months later, while Susan was being dialyzed, her mother informed me that she was expecting another baby. To my great dismay, she admitted that she and Susan's estranged biological father had briefly reconciled when he had come to Pittsburgh. After the baby was born, her mother was confronted with overwhelming responsibilities—another child to feed on top of tending to Susan's increasing health needs and her elderly mother's failing health.

While Susan's mother was on the bus returning from work one late evening, she suddenly developed profuse bleeding per her vagina. The bus driver was compelled to unload the passengers and summon an ambulance. She was brought to a local hospital, where testing revealed that she had inoperable uterine cancer and multiple metastases. She died several days later. I was shocked to find out that she was only thirty-seven years old, yet she looked closer to fifty. Susan had no other relatives and because her grandmother could not take care of the now one-year-old baby as well as Susan and her other brother, Social Services opted to place the children in foster homes. However, street-smart, feisty, resourceful, strong-willed, and determined Susan had a sense of responsibility well beyond her years and convinced her grandmother and Social Services that she, together with her grandmother, can care for her siblings and that Susan could take care of herself. However, despite Susan's praiseworthy intentions and determination to remain independent, this complicated and untenable arrangement failed. About four months later, Susan was brought to our ER with another hypertensive crisis; there, she arrested and died. All her caretakers were heartbroken. Her grandmother died soon after as well. Susan's life had so many elements of a Greek tragedy. I often wonder what the future held for her and what she could have accomplished if she had a supportive family environment.

Dani or Becky: Lack of Parenting and its Long-Term Mental and Physical Health Effects on Children

One cannot overstate the influence of good parenthood and proper upbringing on children's lives. I firmly believe that the interactions of children and their immediate families during the first few years of life forge a largely predictable path that many, though not all, children follow throughout life. I came to this conclusion not through any formal study but by my close personal interactions with and observations of numerous families over the years. Neglect or inadequate emotional support on the part of caretakers can significantly impair the social and physical development of children. Insufficient parental education and lack of financial resources may also contribute to insufficient parenting. Moreover, chronic mental and physical health issues in a parent or in another sibling may further compromise the mental and physical health of all individuals in such stressed households. These factors combine to make what I call a "social incendiary device," the main target of which is the ill child.

Notably, while the physical aspects of disease are usually either visible or measurable by scientific instruments, mental and psychological issues are much more difficult to detect or quantify. The following anecdote illustrates how a lack of emotional nurturing during the formative years can torment children well into adolescence and beyond.

I cared for Dani since her birth on March 1996, through age twenty. I also had the opportunity to observe the short- and-long term effects of poor parenting on her mental health, thereby gaining some insight into Dani's mental and, by extension, physical disorder.

Dani was born prematurely to a seventeen-year-old mother and eighteen-year-old father who were high school sweethearts—as well as high school dropouts with impressive truancy history.

Both parents were physically healthy and handsome, intelligent yet poorly educated, estranged from their families, and without financial resources. Growing up, they quickly learned how to take advantage of all perquisites available to the needy through CHP. They also deftly manipulated the various government agencies and human services, and somehow managed to subsist.

Dani was born prematurely and sustained injury to several organs due to disruption of the placenta resulting in prolonged circulatory failure and reduced oxygen supply to the entire body just before birth, a process known as *asphyxia*. This disorder is a well-recognized harbinger of serious injury to the intestine (*necrotizing enterocolitis*) and to the kidneys (*acute cortical necrosis*), both of which were evident in Dani. As a result, shortly after birth, she required emergency resection of a devitalized portion of her intestine that left her with short gut syndrome and prolonged nutritional difficulties. She also developed permanent and severe kidney failure. This meant that she required dialysis to remain alive after her gastrointestinal surgery. These circumstances essentially rendered me the doctor in charge of all her medical needs.

Although peritoneal dialysis is better tolerated than hemodialysis in infants (see "*Noah's Princess*"), and their parents can be trained to perform this procedure at home with less interruption to their lifestyle, this was not an option in Dani because the surface area of the membrane covering the abdominal wall and intestinal contents was compromised by her prior abdominal surgery. Consequently, I initiated hemodialysis. This procedure presented numerous logistical and technical problems, as described in pp. 23 and 58. Because of her small body size (her birth weight was 6.5 lbs) and loss of large blood vessels that were previously accessed in conjunction with her gastrointestinal procedures, establishing adequate vascular access for hemodialysis became very challenging. Moreover, because of circulatory and blood pressure instability associated with hemodialysis, she had to be admitted and closely monitored in the ICU during each dialysis session. Because my dialysis nurses felt insecure dialyzing such a medically unstable baby, I had to remain in proximity in the ICU to support my team during each four-hour dialysis session over the next twenty-one months. Special transport from her home to CHP ICU was arranged three times per week.

Dani's overall home care also raised concerns because her parents were immature, constantly quarrelling, and unwilling or unable to carry out complex medical guidelines. Thus, Dani's special nutritional requirements were compromised and compliance with proper timing and dosages of several medications was questionable.

A major advantage of seeing Dani so frequently in the ICU was that my nurses and I were able to review and reinforce the medical and nutritional regimens. In addition, because Dani was the only person in the ICU who was not acutely ill, we all invested time socializing with this adorable baby. Indeed, Dani was very responsive, pleasant, and affectionate. After a short period, she would stand up while holding on to the sides of her crib and jump, laugh and mumble words in my direction as soon as I entered the ICU. I and other caretakers were equally excited to see her. Although it was common for me to place emotional energy in bonding with children during my entire career, that expended with Dani was never exceeded.

Because of our collective efforts, Dani thrived. By the time she was twenty-two months old, she was of appropriate length and weighed sixteen pounds. She also exhibited excellent cognitive development. Although her mother rarely accompanied Dani to CHP, we convinced her to become a kidney donor. Apart from the typical potential technical obstacles related to transplantation in younger children, Dani's prior abdominal surgery had restricted her abdominal cavity and made the vascular connections more challenging. Yet, het postoperative progress was surprisingly smooth. Her kidney functioned very well, and there were no major complications. She was discharged to the care of her father, who seemed more invested in her. However, despite the many efforts of our renal Social Service worker and all caregivers to encourage and support the parents, routine visits to the outpatient pediatric renal transplant clinic occurred erratically.

Dani's biological parents had a second child together before they separated permanently when Dani was about four years old. After that, her mother completely vanished from Dani's life. Dani was then under the care of her father and his girlfriend.

While driving to work one morning and listening to the news on the radio, my attention was aroused when I heard the name of Dani's father's in connection with his arrest for child abuse and neglect. Apparently, a neighbor heard the persistent, loud cries of children coming from Dani's trailer and called 911. The police found eight children ranging in age from one to nine years, living in squalid conditions cramped in one of the two rooms of the trailer, together with several malnourished cats. Some children were soiled with feces and had dirty diapers. There was a pile of dirty dishes in the sink, empty cans of processed food in overflowing garbage cans, and an empty refrigerator. These conditions were later depicted on the evening news. Among the eight children was Dani.

The parents returned to the trailer eight hours later, after an excursion at the Meadows Race Track and Casino and were promptly arrested. Apparently, Dani's father had two additional children by different mothers, and his current girlfriend had four children of her own. Children's and Youth Services eventually found foster homes for all eight children, the first of several home placements for Dani. Many of these foster parents looked after other children with medical conditions. The unfortunate reality is that for a few foster parents, this is not an altruistic act but a means of collecting a monthly stipend while providing little emotional support, kindness, or adequate medical and dietary supervision.

Over the ensuing years, Dani exhibited anxiety, tremors, sleep disorders, truancy, and poor school performance. On occasion, she was temperamental. These behavioral problems persisted unabated and made her placement in subsequent foster homes increasingly difficult; these issues endangered her transplanted kidney as well as her overall physical health. She had delayed menarche and sexual development. Her short gut syndrome caused recurrent diarrhea or constipation and a poorly characterized abdominal pain that resulted in many emergency department visits as well as several hospital admissions.

By about twelve years of age, Dani was assigned the psychiatric diagnosis of posttraumatic stress disorder with dissociative identity disorder. As she entered adolescence, her psychiatric admissions became more frequent and prolonged. She had flashbacks, anxiety, and exhibited aggressive and combative behavior. She also had two admissions for suicidal ideation, and several psycho-behavioral agents were tried with variable success. Remarkably, through all these problems spanning many years, including documented periods of poor compliance with her anti-rejection medications, her kidney function remained stable and satisfactory. However, during late adolescence, she became more rebellious and noncompliant, and was eventually treated for two episodes of rejection.

Fortunately, at fourteen years of age, Dani was placed in the foster care of a wonderful woman who truly understood, tolerated, and supported Dani in every possible way. This woman formally adopted Dani when she was seventeen, and to help erase her past, she changed Dani's name to Becky. For the first time in her life, Becky experienced a stable and supportive family environment. Yet, although she seemed outwardly happy and flashed a radiant smile, emotionally, Becky continued to conceal a great deal of pain and anger that still erupted from time to time. It seemed as if her trust and faith in adults had been betrayed for so long and so often that she had difficulty recognizing and accepting true love when it was finally offered. Considering her social history, I believe that Becky's destiny was both predictable and inevitable.

A SPECIAL CASE OF RENAL TRANSPLANTATION

When I first arrived in Pittsburgh, there was no formal renal clinic. Because there were so few successful pediatric renal transplants at that time, these were not offered or performed on a regular basis. This consideration also obviated the use of chronic dialysis that is considered a temporary solution or prelude to transplantation. Chronic dialysis was also discouraged because it was cumbersome, expensive, and both physically and emotionally traumatic, particularly in younger children.

In fact, as noted earlier in, "*Major issues confronting children with chronic renal failure at the start of my nephrology career*," our own well-intentioned psychologist at CHP, Dr. Reinhart, had expressed his opposition to transplantation and, by inference, to dialysis in an editorial in the *Journal of Pediatrics*, claiming that such interventions constituted "a form of torture of children and their families." This view was completely opposite that of the newly arrived junior physician fresh out of fellowship—namely, me. These divergent viewpoints were tested by a challenging high-profile case encountered several months later.

Our highly respected pediatrician Dr. Paul Gaffney invited me to attend the weekly Tumor Board Committee meeting on a Friday afternoon. The discussion centered on a one-and-a-half-year-old girl who, six months earlier, had her left kidney removed because of a malignant mass known as Wilms tumor. She had just been readmitted with recurrence of Wilms in the only remaining kidney, the right kidney, along with a tumor spread or *metastases* to her lungs. The latter caused an accumulation of fluid in the normally narrow space between the lungs and the inner chest wall, or *pleural effusions*, thereby preventing full lung expansion and compromising breathing. She had been started on chemotherapy with actinomycin D but had not responded favorably. The cancer experts informed me that the renal mass was large, and per prior experience, its removal could enhance the management and promote regression of the lung metastases. The specific question posed to me by this committee was: What care options could be offered and could the infant survive if the remaining kidney was removed?

Without any hesitation, I replied, "We will support the child through peritoneal dialysis, and if the metastases resolved and she became disease-free for a year, I would recommend renal transplantation." Several of the senior faculty, including Dr. Reinhart, expressed both surprise and skepticism as to whether I had carefully considered if such interventions could offer a long-term benefit and at what price. However, there was no alternative treatment plan that would offer any chance for survival, so the committee accepted my plan. The child's mother was ecstatic to learn of this decision. As it turned out, mother was healthy, had the same blood type as her daughter, and was willing and eager to become an organ donor. Fortunately, the clinical course was smooth, and the child had an excellent outcome.

The following letter was composed by this patient just after I saw her in my clinic for our last visit together when she was twenty years old; it is one of the most gratifying letters I received throughout my entire career.

Dr. Ellis,   6·20/0

    I am used to giving you candy canes or pictures of how I've grown - those are easy - however, writing a goodbye letter is not only unfamiliar it is also very hard and sad for me to do.

    You have been there even before I could even pronounce the word kidney or understand the word cancer you have always been my "daddy" away from home. As a young child with health issues I could have been scared of the hospital, however, you kept the scariness away. I was (and still am) excited to come to Children's Hospital. I would forget how miserable being poched and prodded with freezing instruments because all I could think about was how excited I was to go see Dr. Ellis.

    Not only did you give me great care as a patient, but you were also a friend and a father-like figure to me as a person. I am twenty years old but still get just as giddy as I did when I was ~~you were~~ younger.

    As you can see you have such an impact in my life and I just want to thank you for all the years and all you have done for me! I can only hope my new doctors and new hospital are half as great as you and the rest of Childrens has been to me! I will miss you dearly!
              Love you!

ANOTHER RENAL TRANSPLANTATION STORY

Because I discuss several aspects of transplantation in various portions of this book and because the information is pertinent to this story, I am compelled to provide the reader with a brief background on this topic.

Prior to 1981, renal transplantation outcomes were generally poor, inconsistent, operator- and center-dependent, fraught with technical complications, and with many deleterious effects stemming from the immunosuppressive agents. Parenthetically, transplantation of other organs was much less successful and largely abandoned. Consequently, before 1981, renal transplants were performed in a few children at a handful of institutions, and they usually involved kidney donation from a parent or older sibling. Apart from technical problems, common side effects of medications included disfigurement, poor linear growth, obesity, diabetes, and hypertension largely related to high-dose steroids, and serious infections attributed to azathioprine use. Indeed, the poor quality of life, at times negated the benefits of transplantation and limited its widespread application. Hence, the availability of a more selective immunosuppressive agent that, in theory, was superior in controlling rejection—and hence improve transplant outcomes while limiting these deleterious, systemic side effects—could revolutionize the field of human transplantation. Preliminary data in adult kidney transplant recipients in England suggested that cyclosporine A (CsA), later renamed "cyclosporine," had such unique properties.

May 1981 marks an important milestone for the University of Pittsburgh, School of Medicine, UPMC, because Dr. Thomas Starzl arrived from Denver, Colorado, to head the newly formed transplantation division. I suspect that his recruitment to Pittsburgh was facilitated by two principal factors. First, Dr. Henry T. Bahnson, who headed the entire surgery department in Pittsburgh, was a long-time friend. Second, Dr. Starzl was just contracted by the National Institutes of Health and Sandoz, which owned the rights to cyclosporine or Sandimmune, to conduct a major clinical trial in the United States, using this agent in any and all transplants. This was a highly anticipated trial, since it offered the prospect of meaningful survival to so many individuals awaiting life-saving transplantation; it could also bring much acclaim and prestige to the University of Pittsburgh. As will become quite evident later in this book, I was not just a witness but also an active participant in this major enterprise.

My interaction with the first pediatric renal transplant recipient to receive cyclosporine was in May 1981. I vividly recall receiving a telephone call directly from Dr. Starzl on a Monday morning. I had become aware that he would oversee all transplant services, including the existing transplant surgery program that, at that time, consisted almost solely of renal transplantation. He wished to forewarn me that a six-year-old Saudi Arabian girl, Amira, who was under his care, would be accompanying him to Pittsburgh. Even though Amira had royal blood she led a nomadic existence in the Saudi Arabian desert. She had end-stage renal disease (ESRD) and required dialysis and transplantation. She was flown by helicopter to Riyadh and from there to Denver. Amira would be arriving at Pittsburgh at seven o'clock that evening, on the same flight as Dr. Strazl. He continued, "Amira's hemodialysis catheter is not functional, so she had not dialyzed for four days and had a low-grade fever." He had a soft voice with a slight southern accent, and a paternalistic overtone toward Amira that made him very persuasive. Dr. Starzl ended his call by saying, "I would consider it a personal favor if you could attend to her promptly upon our arrival."

Late that evening, I met Amira along with her twenty-year-old brother, who had accompanied her. Neither of them could speak English, and unlike later on, we did not have staff to serve as dedicated interpreters. Amira wore a black burqa and was resistant to being touched or examined by me or other male physicians. I obtained cultures of her blood and from the dialysis catheter (*Vascath*) exit site that was oozing purulent material and appeared inflamed. We then administered antibiotics by vein to manage presumed exit site infection followed by de-clotting of the catheter using a strong heparin solution;

she was successfully dialyzed early the following morning. The infection resolved, and the dialysis catheter continued to function well. On June 18, 1981, Amira received a kidney donated by a brain-dead individual and had an exceptionally uneventful postoperative course.

Through a lucrative financial arrangement between the government of Saudi Arabia and UPMC, all medical expenses along with living expenses for Amira were underwritten; a very generous $20,000 a year stipend was also provided to her brother.

In the two years that followed, Amira and her brother became completely acculturated and achieved fluency in conversational English. They were outgoing, pleasant, and generally appeared very happy with their lives. Her brother bought a red convertible sedan and soon after had an American girlfriend. He dressed in colorful shirts and tight pants and enjoyed going to parties. Amira started to wear tight fitting leather pants or blue jeans with intentional holes and worn appearance, as was the style then—I have never seen her wear anything black since then. She became particularly infatuated with and idolized Michael Jackson. It was clear that both she and her brother wanted to prolong their stay in Pittsburgh; resuming a nomadic lifestyle seemed out of the question. By this time, many full-time Arabic interpreters—some of whom were MDs, accountants, and others—closely interacted with the now-flourishing transplant program that serviced nearly all Saudi Arabia. Thus, it was an interpreter who, in May 1983, informed me that because Amira had done well for nearly two years after the transplant, the government requested that she and her brother return to Saudi Arabia. In fact, the interpreter said, "All arrangements are in place for Amira's clinical transition and follow-up care in Riyadh."

When I saw Amira for what was to be her last renal clinic visit in April 1983, she was very distraught because Michael Jackson was performing in Pittsburgh that June and she was due to depart for Saudi Arabia in May. One week prior to her departure, we obtained routine outpatient monitoring renal studies and for the very first time noted a rise in serum creatinine from 0.6 to 1.3. This value signaled an abrupt and significant reduction in kidney function the cause of which was not apparent. However, later that day we discovered that her blood cyclosporine level was undetectable. Other findings included a palpably tender transplanted kidney which upon biopsy confirmed our suspected clinical diagnosis of acute cellular rejection. Confronted with these data, Amira tearfully confessed to stopping the cyclosporine because she did not want to miss the upcoming concert. Fortunately, after appropriate treatment, she overcame the moderate, early rejection. Nevertheless, this acute event protracted her departure from the States, thus enabling her to attend the Michael Jackson concert after all. In fact, Amira and her brother found ingenious ways of prolonging their return to Saudi Arabia for another three years.

THE HEAVY BURDEN OF CHILDREN WITH
DISABILITIES AND SPECIAL NEEDS ON FAMILIES

I have a huge amount of respect and sympathy for families caring for children with special needs and disabilities. About one-half of all children with kidney disorders have coexisting acquired or developmental mental and/or other medical conditions. Many such children have renal and urinary tract disorders with anatomic anomalies often evident on prenatal ultrasound, breathing difficulties surrounding birth, or genetic mutations affecting both the kidneys and other organs. Unlike children with isolated kidney disorders that also require transplantation, the quality of life of children affected by such co-morbidities may not be ameliorated even after successful transplantation. In some of these children and their families, the stress is not confined to the pre-transplant period but may persist and, at times, becomes exacerbated after transplantation. As one may surmise, most of these families do not cope well with the indefinite period of medical uncertainty and emotional stress.

In most children with co-morbidities, the renal component is not severe enough to necessitate dialysis and/or transplantation. Thus, the clinical manifestations of these children vary broadly in severity. In general, however, symptoms and signs tend to occur at a very young age and last for years, sometimes for a lifetime. If the condition is mostly limited to the genitourinary tract and is well managed, in my experience, the family's lifestyle is not disrupted excessively and most such families tend to cope relatively well. However, a small but not trivial fraction of children with these more slowly progressive renal disorders have associated cognitive and developmental impairment and other anomalies, such as trisomy 21, cardiac disease or severe autism. These children truly deserve the designation of "special needs" and often have a major impact on their parents' marriage and the lifestyles of their siblings. Their psychobehavioral problems are often compounded by inadequate family support, education gap, health issues in other family members, financial constraints, rural residence location, and unavailability of social or community support programs. In some cases, these children need constant supervision and are unable to travel away from their immediate geographic location. Thus, the family could never go on vacation. In extreme cases, this is tantamount to being on house arrest. The siblings may also be deprived of the parents' attention, which is mostly directed to the sick child. The parents' concerns often increase, rather than decrease, as their children get older, and they feel great guilt if or when they eventually must relinquish care of their beloved child to "strangers" at an institution. Heather's case exemplifies the tremendous stress that parents endure when they devote so much energy to serve their children with special needs.

I first met Heather as an infant, after she presented with high fever, vomiting, and listlessness. She was quickly diagnosed with a urinary tract infection and responded well to antibiotics. Further testing showed mildly reduced renal function, malformed kidneys on ultrasound, and vesicoureteral reflux, a common dysfunction of the ureter connection to the bladder that predisposes to urinary tract infection (see, "*Precious*"). Nowadays, this constellation of findings falls under the diagnostic umbrella of *congenital anomalies of the kidneys and urinary tract*, or CAKUT. With proper supervision and management,

Heather had very few breakthrough or clinically evident urinary tract infections, and her kidney function remained remarkably stable over the next nearly three decades. However, it became clear early in her life that Heather had severe mental impairment and minimal verbal communication. She was uncooperative and combative which together with an exceptional physical strength made her difficult to handle in clinic. She was an only child to loving parents, and her mother was especially attentive to all her basic needs. Despite her nonexistent social life, her mother never complained.

When I last saw Heather in my clinic, she was nearly thirty years old. Her mother insisted on bringing her to me exclusively, probably because she behaved like a two-year-old and partially because her mother sensed that I had empathy for her daughter, whom I had cared for since birth. Mother always credited me for saving her daughter. After Heather's mother died at a young age, her father came across the following letter his wife had intended to send to me. He wrote:

"Heather and I lost her in March 2006 to the cancer, but I am sure she would want to express her thoughts in the note to you.

Heather continues to maintain good kidney function and is in general good health except for the outbursts which keeps her in a wheelchair most of the time.

I hope that you are well and again say thank you.

Sincerely, S. Rx (Heather's dad)"

5/30/05

Dear Dr. Ellis,

We want to thank you for the wonderful care you have given Heather over these many years.

Your expertise is without question, but your kindness and patience were so important. Heather is not the ideal patient, but you always treated her and me with dignity and compassion. You have been our "security blanket" for almost 30 years and we will miss you.

God bless you.

With our best wishes and affection,

Mr. and Mrs. —— and of course, Heather

Sub-specialization

HYPERTENSION (HTN OR HIGH BLOOD PRESSURE)

FOR AS LONG as I can remember, I have had a special interest in hypertension. Although this condition is more common in children than most people realize, it had received little attention prior to 1980. The list of conditions associated with hypertension in children is perhaps even more extensive than in adults and includes numerous rare genetic or congenital disorders. The clinical presentation of hypertension is also quite variable depending on the child's age. Consequently, I approached the detection of these causes in a detective-like manner. I could not resist the challenge of deciphering these conditions that sometimes manifested clinically in the first day of life and extended through childhood. Management of hypertension is also very challenging in children. In the early part of my career, there were few agents available for managing hypertension in adults, and even fewer that could be used in children. Dosage guidelines were often extrapolated from adult data using age and body size, and not supported by fact-based studies of drug efficacy and safety in children. Thus, in contrast to adults, who typically have multifactorial or primary hypertension, the evaluation of hypertensive children is much more complex and challenging and management tends to be more individualized.

Because kidney disorders account for most of the causes of hypertension in preadolescent and non-obese children, pediatric nephrologists have traditionally assumed a key role in evaluating and managing these children. This in sharp contrast to most hypertensive adults that are managed by cardiologists or internists. In fact, for a long time, I was one of a handful of pediatricians involved in studies assessing the benefits of antihypertensive agents in children, and I published several articles on the topic. For these efforts, in 1999, the American Society of Hypertension awarded me with a certificate, recognizing me as a hypertension specialist—I proudly displayed this on my office wall. In addition, I was invited to contribute review articles on this subject, the latest of which appeared in the prestigious textbook *Pediatric Nephrology* in 2016 (Avner ED et al., Eds, Springer Press, 6th edition, 2015, pp. 1541-1576). The following are selected anecdotes related to hypertension that you may find interesting and informative.

PHEOCHROMOCYTOMA

Very few hypertensive disorders are as enigmatic or intriguing in their clinical presentation as pheochromocytoma. Less than one year into my career, I encountered my very first referral. He was a nine-year-old Amish boy, the middle of eight siblings, who suffered from headache and dizziness. He visited a local family physician who found his blood pressure to be markedly elevated. This discovery was fortuitous because, in those days, measuring a child's blood pressure was uncommon even among pediatricians. A large tumor was discovered on ultrasound of the adrenal glands, a predilection site for this tumor. This finding, together with a high urinary excretion of vanillylmandelic acid, supported my presumptive diagnosis of *pheochromocytoma*, or *pheo*. When I screened his asymptomatic siblings for hypertension, I found it in four. They also had similar proof of adrenal pheos. In this disorder, hypertension arises from secretion of large quantities of epinephrine (adrenaline) and/or norepinephrine (noradrenaline) secreted by the tumor cells, not in response to a physiologic stimulus, such as exercise or a fall in blood pressure, but at rest. These hormones cause marked vascular wall constriction and occasional rise in pulse, resulting in hypertension. They are metabolized in the body and excreted in the urine as vanillylmandelic acid that serves as a screening test for this disorder. All abnormalities resolve after tumor removal. However, there were several reports of lethal complications in adults related to acute rises in blood pressure during surgical manipulation of the tumor. This complication could be avoided or minimized by proper preoperative preparation of the patient. In addition, low blood pressure—hypotension—can cause dizziness and syncope after tumor removal. There was limited information in the medical literature concerning the intraoperative management of pheos in children. Confronted with this child and his siblings, I devised a medical protocol designed to manage the hypertension preoperatively and prevent the development of hypotension postoperatively. After I utilized this approach successfully in eight consecutive children, I published our experience in a reputable pediatric journal (Ellis D. and Gartner J.C. The intraoperative medical management of childhood pheochromocytoma. *J. Pediatr. Surg.* 15:65, 1980). I am happy to report that with minor modifications this approach is still widely utilized today.

Notably, after discovering pheos in the above patient and his siblings, I offered to measure the blood pressure in their forty-five-year-old father. He denied experiencing any of the several hypertension signs and symptoms that I had reviewed with each of his children and boasted that he was capable of intense labor on his farm for up to sixteen hours a day without fatigue or other complaints. Indeed, he was a strong man with hands that were hypertrophied and heavily calloused, attesting to his physical workload. He reluctantly consented to have his blood pressure taken—it was markedly elevated at 240/130 mmHg, and his pulse was fifty beats per minute. I then contacted a colleague at the adjoining Presbyterian University Hospital, who promptly diagnosed him with a very large pheo that was removed uneventfully two weeks later. This colleague had previously published a study on

140 adults with pheochromocytomas that he had discovered during mass screening of multiple Amish families attending an annual family reunion in rural Pennsylvania. He recognized the name of the patient I referred to him—he belonged to the same family tree.

Over the ensuing decades, I encountered many other children with HTN caused by pheos. Most, but not all, had a genetic or familial predisposition for this tumor, which is largely morphologically benign in terms of pathology, but can be clinically fatal if not appropriately managed. One such case was a teenager referred to me directly from a dental office. Despite being asymptomatic, he was markedly hypertensive and was at high risk of developing an acute hypertensive crisis if certain anesthetic agents had been administered prior to the routine dental procedure. In my experience, the detection of hypertension by a dentist is quite rare, and I commended him for discovering this disorder. It turned out that this pheo was of the rare malignant type. Fortunately, the tumor was localized, rather than spread to distant parts of the body, and was removed without complications.

Two other children had unique clinical presentations that illustrate the elusive nature of pheos. The first was a five-year-old male born to a healthy, young couple. In 1983, he was admitted to his local hospital because of unexplained tremors and agitation. Other less concerning symptoms included diminished appetite and feeling somewhat fatigued or less active. These presenting symptoms are rare at that age. A drug toxicology screen was negative, and at eleven p.m. the following day, I received a call from his admitting physician who had been summoned to see the child because of increased severity of his symptoms and because his blood pressure, which had been normal on admission, was now quite high, at 135/80 mmHg. I arranged for immediate transport to CHP, and I arrived at our Emergency Department just prior to his arrival by ambulance.

On examination, the boy was very thin, extremely agitated, and trembling. Given his age, the blood pressure was now even higher—150/90 mmHg. He was admitted directly to the intensive care unit where I contemplated the cause and, more importantly, treatment for impending hypertensive encephalopathy, which could manifest with more severe neurologic symptoms, such as seizures, coma, or stroke. Based on the severity of his symptoms, I suspected a pheo. When I inquired into the family history of hypertension and, specifically of pheo, the young parents were unaware of any hypertensive relatives but promised to check with their parents after getting back home. The boy's symptoms were so prominent that I decided to do a test for presumptive presence of pheo using an intravenous agent—phentolamine. A rapid lowering of blood pressure in response to this unique agent is prima fascia evidence for pheo. Within two minutes of receiving a minute dosage of phentolamine, there was a precipitous fall in blood pressure to 70/40 mmHg. Although his agitation and trembling immediately resolved, I was concerned about the abrupt drop in blood pressure. Fortunately, it quickly normalized after I administered a saline fluid bolus by vein. Again, the initial urine studies and subsequent abdominal ultrasound were consistent with pheo. After transitioning to my now published pheo protocol, the blood pressure became controlled, and the tumor was uneventfully removed three weeks later.

Notably, on the day after transfer of their son to CHP, I met up with the parents who presented me with a laminated article published in Washington, D.C., in 1958. The article described how a large adrenal tumor was successfully removed from a markedly hypertensive midshipman, the boy's uncle, during a "fifteen-hour marathon operation" at Walter Reed Army Hospital; this proved to be a benign pheo.

Another memorable pheo presentation took place in late evening just prior to Christmas in 1989. I was asked to do an urgent consultation for hypertension in a fifteen-year-old female who had just been transported to the CHP ICU in an unresponsive state. Apparently, the teenager was in good health but had had a verbal confrontation with her mother because she was not permitted to go to a party with her boyfriend. Reluctantly, she remained home, and after calming down, she eventually helped her mother make Christmas cookies. She went to bed around 1:00 a.m. On the following morning, she did not come down for breakfast; her parents assumed that she had simply slept late because she was on holiday break. At about noon, they decided to wake her up but found her unresponsive. The paramedics were then notified and after a brief interval at a local emergency department, she was transferred directly to the CHP ICU. Given her lack of a preexisting medical disorder together with the quarrel with her mother on the previous evening, we suspected that she had attempted suicide, possibly by drug overdose. Hence, the initial diagnostic studies included a comprehensive toxicology screen and biochemical and hematologic studies, all of which were unrevealing. In the meantime, she remained in a coma without a clear cause. A computerized tomography (CT) scan on her brain and other imaging studies of the chest and abdomen were done that disclosed a large tumor above the right kidney, within the adrenal gland. The CT also showed swelling in the posterior part of the brain, raising suspicion of posterior reversible encephalopathy syndrome. Thus, it became apparent that the above interpersonal family circumstances had briefly diverted us from suspecting severe hypertensive encephalopathy, or brain involvement, secondary to possible pheo. Within two hours of arriving at our ICU, arrangements were made to remove the tumor. However, on transport from the ICU to the operating room, she had a cardiorespiratory arrest, and despite immediate and appropriate intervention, she could not be resuscitated. This was a tragic loss. On autopsy, the tumor proved to be a benign pheo.

HAS DEMETRI GONE APE?

By all accounts, Samantha was an extraordinary representative of her species. She was intelligent, energetic, affectionate, playful, and socially interactive. Perhaps she was even good-looking, although, as the saying goes, beauty is in the eye of the beholder. No wonder she had endeared herself to all her caretakers ever since she and her cousin Melvin had arrived as infants at the Pittsburgh Zoo from the Republic of the Congo. Her ear-to-ear smile was infectious, and despite exposing very large and sharp teeth, Samantha was hardly intimidating or frightening. She enjoyed her connection, particularly to very young children who came to visit her repeatedly and appeared to engage them in unintelligible conversation. In short, as a chimpanzee, Samantha displayed a high order of intelligence and humanlike behavior. Therefore, it would be a gross injustice to mistake Samantha—an ape— for a monkey; this would be highly disrespectful and insulting to her.

I first met Samantha in 1983 by way of her illness. She was a fully-grown but chronologically young seven-years old when she first developed symptoms consisting of gradual loss of appetite and body weight, as well as reduced activity level. Her caretakers became increasingly concerned, particularly since Melvin had started to exhibit similar unexplained symptoms about two months later. After several calls to various other zoos in the United States, the zookeeper became informed that many chimps from the same geographic origin of the Congo had developed similar symptoms and died unexpectedly within a year. Furthermore, the veterinarians at the Miami Zoo had discovered that chimps they had received from the same colony as Samantha had elevated blood pressure and mild to moderate renal failure. Notably, several autopsies had revealed diffuse small vessel (*arteriolar*) disease of the kidneys. Together, these findings pointed to a primary renal disorder, but the underlying cause of the pathologic findings was not apparent. The heart and other organs seemed unaffected, and renal ultrasound studies were suspiciously abnormal but inconclusive. Shortly thereafter, Samantha and her cousin underwent sedation to help obtain accurate blood pressure measurements and were found to have very high blood pressure (160/95 mmHg); renal function was also reduced in both.

After a brief review of the veterinary and medical literature, the local zoo veterinarian came across my name in conjunction with several publications related to renal vascular disease, such as renal artery stenosis, which is a relatively common cause of hypertension in younger children. Because of this and because of the reduced kidney function in Samantha, he called me at my office. He gave me a medical synopsis of Samantha and asked my advice. I informed him that I had very limited experience with hypertension in animals other than research I had done involving the spontaneously hypertensive rat (Ellis D, Banner B, Janosky JE, Feig PU: Potassium supplementation attenuates experimental hypertensive renal injury in rats. J Am Soc Nephrol 2:1529-1537, 1992). In this animal model of hypertension, dietary supplementation with potassium reduced systemic blood pressure and protected against kidney injury by ameliorating small vessel disease present within the kidneys of these rats. These findings could only remotely pertain to Samantha's condition. A more plausible explanation was that a hereditary predilection, together with an environmental trigger, possibly dietary or infectious, may have initiated the renal disorder that then caused the hypertension. I confessed that I really had little idea of how to go about proving this hypothesis. However, my curiosity kicked. So, I suggested implementing an abbreviated protocol to help evaluate the suspected renal vascular etiology, as I would have done in a young child. I also requested borrowing the pathologic slides from Miami, so my expert pathologist at CHP, Dr. Eduardo Yunis, and I could review the findings.

When Samantha's laboratory results became available one week later, they were consistent with mild renal functional impairment and high circulating plasma levels of the hormone renin, which derives from the kidneys and can cause systemic hypertension. Urinalysis revealed an elevated amount of urinary protein that can also occur in renal microvascular causes of hypertension; there were no other urinary abnormalities. Our independent review of the biopsy slides from Miami suggested mild to moderate small vessel wall thickening (*intimal hyperplasia*) without any inflammatory component or fibrinoid necrosis to suggest a vasculitis. When I discussed these findings with the zoo veterinarian, I again expressed my reluctance to become further involved in Samantha's management because I did not feel confident in conceiving an effective scientifically-based management plan. However, I had already invested a good deal of time, and I was moved by the extraordinary love and concern the zoo personnel had shown for Samantha. I also thought of all the other chimps that were in peril. So, when prompted about further testing or treatment, I mentioned that aortic and renal angiography may be useful in assessing the kidney vessels before considering treatment (possibly using the then newly available agent captopril).

Shortly after suggesting renal angiography, I realized that I was speaking hypothetically and that it was impractical, if not impossible, to perform this highly specialized, complex, and invasive procedure on Samantha. In brief, this procedure begins with powerful sedation or anesthesia. Then, a vascular radiologist, assisted by several technicians, advances an appropriately sized catheter from the femoral artery in the groin, into the aorta, and then into the main renal artery. After ascertaining the catheter location by fluoroscopy, a special liquid, or radio-contrast, is then injected. Because this liquid remains inside the renal vessels for several minutes and outlines the vessels on X-ray films, it can detect narrowing in the larger renal vessels and their branches, while abnormalities in smaller vessels are less distinct. The kidneys eventually excrete this liquid. Given these complexities, there were no veterinary facilities in the Pittsburgh area equipped to perform angiography on Samantha at that time, and certainly no animals were ever evaluated within a private hospital setting.

Here is where the story gets more interesting. After the zoo veterinarian painstakingly obtained several additional blood pressure measurements, he informed me of an incremental trend. I could sense his concern and his passionate plea for urgent action. Hence, I summoned the nerve to contact the vascular radiologist at PUH, who conducted the renal angiography in my patients. Although he principally evaluated adult patients, Dr. Klaus Bron was technically excellent, even with my smallest patients, who were roughly Samantha's weight (about 15 kg). I had a very good rapport with him, and he was always very approachable. I provided Dr. Bron with Samantha's clinical details. After I finished my synopsis, there was a brief silence, possibly because of disbelief at what I was tacitly requesting of him. However, instead of an emphatic no, with relatively little hesitation, and in a calm and reassuring tone, he said he would look into it and call me back.

Hours later, I received his call. He began by stating that going through with this procedure violated several rules, including the unauthorized use of hospital facilities. Therefore, this was a somewhat risky career move for both of us; nonetheless, he had devised a plan that involved bringing Samantha to the hospital after patient hours, smuggling her through a back door and into the radiology department vascular suite. As the head of the vascular radiology service, Dr. Bron had the respect and power to carry out this plan. Thus, he persuaded several loyal assistants to volunteer their services after hours to this clandestine mission. When I explained the general plan to the zoo staff, their excitement at the prospect of gaining any information that could benefit Samantha was palpable. They agreed to administer the sedation.

At 7:00 p.m. on Wednesday that week, Samantha was brought to the designated door of PUH accompanied by the vet and two human parental surrogates. She was alert, somewhat bewildered, but generally well behaved and calm. As planned, she was sedated, spread out on the radiology table, and secured in place. I then did a brief physical examination. When I conducted an ophthalmologic exam to detect hypertensive retinopathy, I was in proximity to Samantha's mouth and was taken aback by her disgusting, malodorous breath that easily penetrated my face mask. Her teeth were large, sharp, and dangerously close to my nose. There was no sign of cardiac abnormality, and her peripheral pulses were strong. An electrocardiogram was done, and then Dr. Bron confirmed the high blood pressure by direct measurement through an intra-arterial transducer introduced into the aorta via the femoral artery. He then methodically and efficiently performed the angiography and obtained excellent images. Although there was a delay in uptake of the radiocontrast medium and a non-discrete blush suggestive of an underlying microvascular disease corresponding to the pathologic findings seen in Miami, no distinct larger vessel anomalies were seen. Samantha tolerated the sedation well and the procedure was successfully completed. I then started Samantha on captopril at a dosage that I extrapolated from human data. By that point, I felt that I had delved deep into the ape business.

Based on blood pressure updates provided to me by the dedicated team at the zoo, there was a good response to captopril. However, to our great disappointment, renal function continued to decline and eventually led to Samantha's death. All her caretakers and admirers, including me, sorely missed her. To my great dismay, despite medical intervention, we also failed to halt the disease progression in Melvin, and he died prematurely.

TEACHING: FROM STUDENT TO EDUCATOR

TEACHING MEDICAL STUDENTS, pediatric residents, and renal fellows is mandatory and constitutes a major yet often under-appreciated component of academic medicine. However, I never considered the experience of teaching as a chore but rather as a great source of inspiration stimulation, empowerment and, ultimately, of my overall professional fulfilment. To effectively impart knowledge on any topic one must first become a diligent student as to master and remain up-to-date with the scientific information. One must then become creative in making the topic as interesting and fun for the student as possible as well as transmit information in the context of one's clinical experience and perspective. Personally, I make a concerted effort to provide concrete and relevant examples of the utility of the information in people's lives because this was a key factor promoting my own motivation when learning from others. Thus, effective teaching extends beyond imparting information; more importantly, it leads to acquisition of knowledge which enables one to make informed as well as meaningful and sensible clinical decisions. Besides underscoring my conviction that basic sciences are central to the understanding of diseases, the sequential process of learning, teaching and reflection of scientific facts and medical concepts acted as a spark igniting my creativity and imagination such that, on occasion, generated an unanticipated level of enlightenment and discovery. I believe that this scenario is largely depicted in the anecdote, *The kidney: "quintessence of form-structure and function"* (p. 121). When these circumstances prevail, one is overcome by tremendous euphoria and excitement, such as that induced by a surge of dopamine or many endorphins, that one wishes to reenact repeatedly. Hence, albeit very demanding, my time commitment and effort invested in the process of teaching has always been emotionally rewarding.

During the first two decades of my career, I had the privilege of participating in the second-year medical student course titled *Preparation to Clinical Medicine*. I contributed to the nephrology curriculum to a modest degree. This course was integrated and coordinated with the basic science curriculum that also included renal pathology as well as biochemistry, physiology, and pharmacology pertinent to the kidney. Students were expected to learn a vast amount of information on each organ system within a relatively brief time ranging from four to six weeks. The class also participated in small-group workshops, where realistic patient vignettes were presented with the aim of demonstrating the clinical or practical application of the material discussed during the formal lectures. Of course, exams and quizzes were given regularly to test the student's knowledge. After the first year, the medical students also had direct involvement with patients in our hospital clinics and in the wards under the supervision of nephrologists such as myself. My interactions with these bright and impressionable students were a welcome opportunity to spark their enthusiasm for this amazing organ, in the same manner that my own professors had inspired me. Unfortunately, because my nephrology division experienced workforce shortages at various times during my career, I had to relinquish my teaching duties at the medical school, first temporarily and, eventually, permanently. It was one of the most regrettable and disappointing aspects of my career.

Another important component of teaching at CHP occurred during my daily supervision of medical care provided to our patients in conjunction with the renal fellows during their inpatient rotations and in the outpatient renal clinic. In addition to formal lectures and informal discussions on many nephrologic topics, I also taught them how to obtain and organize the essential elements of a patient evaluation and how to document the information in a manner that reflected our combined patient assessment. This is very important because the evaluations become part of the permanent patient record, and as the physician on record, I am ultimately responsible for the content of any documentation in the patient record. Yet this vital process is not emphasized enough or formally taught as part of their curriculum. To accomplish this, I had to first dismantle any preconceived notions or defective writing habits. To my great satisfaction, by the end of their fellowship, nearly everyone progressed from writing evaluations with multiple corrections, to no corrections at all.

I also had the opportunity to teach many fourth-year medical students and pediatric residents who elected to take a one-month renal elective. Several promising students chose to apply to our pediatric nephrology training program, and it was gratifying for me to receive thank-you letters from many of them, such as the examples shown below.

Dr. Ellis,   August 23, 2012

    Thank you for making my rotation on Nephrology especially great! I learned so much this month and gained a diverse exposure to Pediatric Nephrology. I really appreciated your willingness to teach and answer all of my questions. I especially appreciated all of the valuable insight and wisdom you shared with me about patient care and medicine. Thanks again!

                    - Lacey ▓▓▓▓in

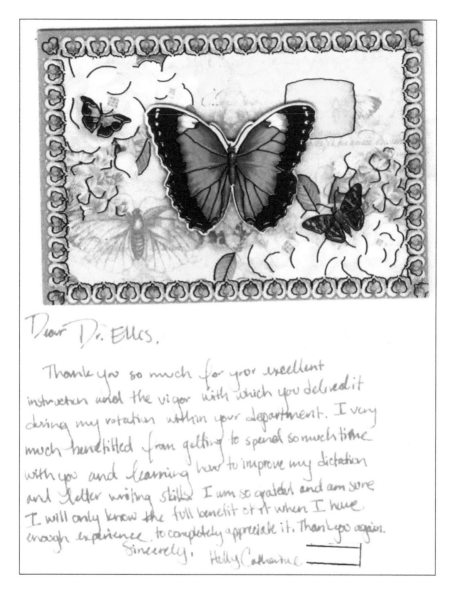

Dear Dr. Ellis,

Thank you so much for your excellent instruction and the vigor with which you delivered it during my rotation within your department. I very much benefitted from getting to spend so much time with you and learning how to improve my dictation and letter writing skills. I am so grateful and am sure I will only know the full benefit of it when I have enough experience to completely appreciate it. Thank you again.

Sincerely, Holly Catharine ————

I am most grateful to all the students and colleagues who valued my commitment to teaching and shared my enthusiasm for learning. Indeed, receiving the coveted Teacher of the Year Award at CHP on two separate occasions were major highlights of my career. Teaching excellence is also a critical component of the Howard Mermelstein Award for Excellence in Pediatrics, and I am privileged to have my name included in the short list of renowned recipients of this award. My selection as the recipient of the National Kidney Foundation Legacy of Leadership Award, in 2018, also serves as affirmation of my entire career in pediatric nephrology. Moreover, in recognition of my teaching contributions, the department of pediatrics at Children's Hospital of Pittsburgh of UPMC established the Demetrius Ellis Annual Lecture in 2013. Thus far, notable invited speakers have included Drs. Ellis Avner, Michelle Baum, Samir S. El-Dahr, Craig Langman, and Minnie Sarwal. Along with the university flier advertising the lecture and the speaker's background and credits, the following summary of my own career is also included:

"Dr. Demetrius Ellis emigrated from Greece at the age of 13 and went on to realize the American dream by becoming a pediatrician. He completed his residency at Children's Hospital of Pittsburgh, and then returned to Pittsburgh after his Renal Fellowship to establish the Pediatric Nephrology Division in 1977.

During his four decades of service, Dr. Ellis relentlessly aspired to exceed his own high clinical, teaching, and research expectations. The foundation of his legacy rests on setting the standard of excellence in clinical care and serving as a passionate and inspirational teacher, role model, and mentor to pediatric residents and the new generation of nephrologists. For fully realizing these key priorities, he has received many Patient Service Awards and the coveted Teacher of the Year Award at CHP on two occasions. Similarly, the medical and alumni staff of CHP recognized him by conferring the Howard A. Mermelstein Award for Excellence in Pediatrics, CHP's highest honor.

Dr. Ellis has published over 150 peer review articles and over 50 book chapters. He has conducted seminal research in the areas of pediatric transplantation, hypertension, and diabetic nephropathy. In fact, many innovative approaches for managing children with kidney transplants and several chronic renal disorders were pioneered by him and are still utilized globally. For these significant accomplishments and for being a founder and pioneer of the field of Pediatric Nephrology, he has been twice nominated for the Henry Barnett Prize which is the highest award conferred by the American Society of Pediatric Nephrology. In addition, the National Kidney Foundation awarded him the prestigious Gift of Life Award in 1993 and the Legacy of Leadership Award on March 10, 2018.

This lecture series celebrates Dr. Ellis' exemplary dedication and effort to improve the health of children with renal disorders in our region."

I was most surprised and privileged to receive a commendation or citation from President George H.W. Bush and both Pennsylvania senators also (not shown) on being honored with the Gift of Life Award by the National Kidney Foundation in 1993.

THE WHITE HOUSE

WASHINGTON

March 16, 1990

Dear Dr. Ellis:

Barbara and I were delighted to learn that you are a recipient of the National Kidney Foundation of Western Pennsylvania's "Gift of Life" award. You have served and inspired others by your generosity and hard work. I am pleased to commend you for your efforts.

With warm regards,

Sincerely,

Geo Bush

Demetrius Ellis, M.D.
Pittsburgh, Pennsylvania

My interest in education is also evident by the publication of over fifty chapters and reviews in leading pediatric nephrology journals and texts. I am particularly proud of my recent comprehensive review on the management of pediatric hypertension based on an understanding of pathophysiology of various disorders published in the textbook *Pediatric Nephrology* (Avner ED et al., Eds, Springer Press, 6th edition, 2015, pp. 1541-1576).

TEACHING ANECDOTES

In my opinion, communication skills are essential for one to become an effective teacher, and the same tools are also critical for interacting with patients and families. These skills are just as important as professional expertise and knowledge. Since most physicians have little formal training in communication, these skills must be learned and refined over time. Of course, some individuals possess more talent in this regard than others. A younger faculty member in my nephrology division was particularly adept at formal speaking. The qualities that he embodied are noted below and served as a template for my own presentations.

TO GIVE OR NOT TO GIVE THE MIKE TO EA

After being the sole pediatric nephrologist at CHP for two years, the chairman of pediatrics and I agreed that we needed to recruit a second staff nephrologist. At that time, CHP was well recognized for its excellent clinical and residency programs. However, the city of Pittsburgh still had a reputation for being a dark, polluted, industrial steel town with an old and outdated pediatric hospital, and a new and small pediatric nephrology component consisting of a single young nephrologist—me. Even after factoring in the low cost of living in Pittsburgh, the salary was also on the low end of the scale.

These circumstances reduced our chances of recruiting one of the very few nephrology fellows graduating from the handful of existing training programs in the United States at that time, or of enticing a more senior pediatric nephrologist to join us. However, to my great surprise, I did receive an application from Dr. Ellis Avner, a graduate of the acclaimed Children's Hospital of Boston's Pediatric Nephrology Fellowship program, at Harvard School of Medicine. On top of this prestigious background, EA was a graduate of Pennsylvania University School of Medicine and Princeton University before that. His academic credentials and research accomplishments were equally impressive. I was reluctant to even contact this upcoming superstar, who was certain to be courted by many centers in more desirable geolocations, with better research facilities and financial support, and salary and compensation packages that we simply could not match. To my astonishment however, EA was excited to hear from me and expressed a genuine interest in the position.

During our initial telephone conversation, it was apparent that he was homesick and wished to return to Pittsburgh. His plan was to bring his wife and raise their future children in the Squirrel Hill neighborhood, where he had lived and attended school as a child. After a couple enthusiastic interviews in person, it became clear that there was good chemistry between us, and very soon after, EA accepted the job offer; he did not even object to the paltry salary.

Within one week of starting his job, I accompanied EA to the main university-affiliated hospital, Presbyterian University Hospital, which still serves as the main hospital facility of what is currently known as the University of Pittsburgh Medical Center (UPMC), where renal grand rounds took place each Wednesday. I gave him a brief preview of the faculty members he was about to meet. Further, I explained the grand-rounds format. Once each month, I shared a pediatric case with this group and discussed various clinical topics of mutual interest, while challenging adult cases were presented on the other three Wednesdays. After the case discussion, diagnostic and management suggestions were solicited from several experienced senior staff physicians. This provided both a great teaching opportunity for younger physicians and a practical patient management forum.

Upon arrival at the conference room, I proudly introduced my new associate to all my colleagues. After the case discussion ended, as usual, the microphone was passed from one senior physician to the next. When the microphone came to EA, to my surprise, he eagerly grabbed it and, with the confidence of a seasoned professor, proceeded to give an eloquent and thorough assessment relating to the complex adult case presented that day. Although questions from junior faculty were encouraged at grand rounds, this was unprecedented. With this sensational debut, it became quite apparent to everyone present that EA was well informed, capable of sound thinking, and articulate. These traits served him well throughout his career.

After his impressive debut at grand rounds, I commended EA on his contribution to the discussion; however, I also mentioned to him that by monopolizing the microphone, he may have done a disservice to the patient under discussion, since there had been no time left for other experts to offer their management suggestions. EA was embarrassed, apologized, and confessed not realizing that he had spoken for such a great length of time. He then thanked me for bringing this issue to his attention and requested I give him a signal if he spoke excessively in the future.

For many years after this encounter, whenever EA spoke at any professional event that I happen to attend, he would periodically glance at me; if I made the familiar "zip it" sign by discreetly dragging my thumb and index fingers across my lips, he would promptly end his speech.

This incident could have been easily forgotten except for the fact that it actually proved a prelude to the development of one of the top nephrology speakers for the next thirty-five years. Within a very short time, EA had perfected and advanced public speaking and lecturing into an art form. He combined his natural charisma of retaining large amounts of written and verbal information with a loud, clear and easy-to-listen voice. His distinct cadence and clear articulation were inimitable. He then honed other skills, including organization and creative and easy-to-understand slides that helped maintain the listeners' interest and focus even when he presented complex scientific concepts. At times, he was inclined to humorous exaggeration and his imagination went a bit wild, but even then, his humor added a unique flavor to his talks. All these qualities and talents combined to make EA an extremely effective speaker, orator and debater, and facilitated his rapid rise in academic medicine. His legacy is truly unparalleled, and I am most grateful that our careers became interwoven when we were budding nephrologists.

Above all else, I value EA's friendship. Although he chose to refer to me as "boss," our friendship was forged first and foremost by mutual respect born out of our shared commitment to providing the highest quality of clinical care with compassion. We were also of similar ages and shared similar lifestyles, raising our young children and having strong, understanding, and supportive wives who also continue to be close friends to this day.

THE KIDNEY: "QUINTESSENCE OF FORM-STRUCTURE AND FUNCTION"

Because of my strong interest and deep commitment to medical education, I remained generally well informed of the modifications and updates in the renal curriculum at the medical school and the limits of the students' fund of information, as well as that of the residents and renal fellows. A strong foundation on basic sciences is invaluable but is relatively useless unless one can apply it to effectively diagnose and treat patients. It was incumbent upon me and other clinicians to help them make this important transition. To accomplish this task, I found it most useful to discuss major kidney concepts, review the pertinent basic science information, and demonstrate how this information was pertinent to the patient whose disease details prompted the discussion. Through personal experience, I came to realize that apart from my open and genuine enthusiasm for all renal topics, interjecting humor contributed to my effectiveness in transmitting medical information and often fostered a greater appreciation and interest in my specialty. I believe that the following anecdote exemplifies several of the concepts contained in the teaching toolbox described in this paragraph.

To introduce the concept of the kidney being the quintessence -prototype- of form-structure and function, I asked the following question: Why is the kidney, kidney bean-shaped or, simply, kidney-shaped? I was quite certain that few, if any students or physicians had ever been asked this question before. Moreover, no one could look this up in the internet where, surely, all answers were to be found. Thus, invariably, my question provoked whimsical smiles and perplexed expressions, without sensible answers.

To answer this question, one must know three basic facts. One, the number of individual functional kidney units, or *nephrons*; two, the physiological functions of the different portions of these nephrons and how they are anatomically organized as to enable the kidney to control the amount of urine production under varying degrees of hydration; and three, the fact that a spherical geometric form or shape can more compactly accommodate the maximum number of nephron units while simultaneously optimizing their ergonomic properties. In fact, the filtering portions of the nephron, the small balls of capillaries called *glomeruli*, reside on the perimeter of the sphere, while the elongated urine producing segments, the tubules and collecting ducts, traverse down toward the center of the sphere. While the first fact could be recalled from anatomy lectures, and the second was stressed in the physiology lecture on the renal countercurrent multiplier system, the answer to why the "kidney is bean-shaped or kidney-shaped" structure was still elusive to my students. This question served as a springboard to reviewing kidney embryology, emphasizing how progenitor cells coalesce into a round mass that eventually gives rise to mature kidneys; for added emphasis, I also mentioned that the kidneys of whales resembled bowling balls. With some imagination, it is easy to view our own "bean-shaped" kidneys as slightly open spheres with a central area, or *renal pelvis*, for the urine to collect before it makes its way down the ureters and into bladder. The sphere is also compressed a bit, so it can fit securely and snuggly in the limited retroperitoneal body location without protruding awkwardly into the abdomen.

After I gave what I thought to be a convincing practical and teleologically sound answer to my question, as a bonus, I asked my students if they could recall the mathematical equation for the volume of a sphere. Of course, all my students had learned this formula at some point along their education, but only a renal fellow with a mechanical engineering degree before entering medical school, Tennille W., exclaimed without hesitation, "$V=4/3\pi r^3$."

Does this story have clinical implications or merely reflects my resounding endorsement of employing an informal, interesting, fun and perhaps creative style of teaching? Indeed, the background information presented thus far served only as a prelude for achieving the primary objective of nearly all my teaching endeavors: relating the facts to patient care. To accomplish this connection, I need to take this story one step further. The above mathematical formula predicts the following: assuming that a healthy adult kidney has a spherical shape with a radius of 2 inches, reducing the radius by just 25 percent reduces its volume by 58 percent. This begs the question, what is the relationship between kidney volume and kidney function? It turns out that kidney size and function are closely related. Admittedly, however, kidney damage and kidney size may not correlate well depending on the specific disease causing progressive nephron injury such that volume loss due to damaged nephrons may be offset by infiltration of inflammatory cells, scar tissue or cysts. Moreover, the rate of deterioration of overall renal function is also variable because we have a second kidney on reserve and because nature has endowed our nephrons with intricate mechanisms that enable them to augment their work load, thus conferring considerable but not unlimited capacity to compensate for the loss of function due to damaged nephrons. Notwithstanding these potential modifiers, the actual volume occupied by the relatively preserved nephrons does decline and as their compensatory limits are exceeded, kidney function deteriorates exponentially rather linearly, such that a patient's very survival may suddenly depend on dialysis or transplantation. Conversely, this hypothesis predicts that measures that can slow down renal injury even to a seemingly small degree, offer the prospect of delaying or perhaps avoiding the need for such drastic, invasive, and expensive interventions. After emphasizing these important concepts, I am finally able to end the discussion by suggesting several patient-specific scientifically-tested practical measures capable of slowing down the rate of renal injury, including lifestyle changes, blood pressure regulation, limiting the amount of protein loss in the urine, managing infection or inflammation in the kidneys through appropriate agents, avoiding nephrotoxic medications, etc.

Although not yet tested, this story led me to hypothesize that similar pathophysiologic considerations apply to other spherical organs exposed to injury. Consequently, a loss in brain cortex of just a couple millimeters can have profound effects on mental function, or small decreases in the radius of thyroid glands, ovaries or testes and a fall in circulating levels of thyroxin, estrogen and testosterone below compensatory levels, respectively, can lead to body-wide metabolic disturbances.

Indeed, in my view, this story truly captures the spirit of teaching and reveals one of my most fundamental sources of inspiration, invigoration, jubilation, and overall professional satisfaction.

PATIENT EDUCATION: MY KIDNEY, MY HERO

As noted in the introduction to, "*Musical Teeth*," the kidney has multiple functions. When renal failure becomes advanced, specific dietary modifications together with medications are commonly employed as to prevent or limit the detrimental clinical manifestations associated with fluid retention or molecular imbalance. These regimens are particularly difficult to enforce in children for several reasons. First, many children are resilient and generally do not feel or act sick despite having diet-related biochemical alterations. This lowers their motivation to change their dietary habits. Second, many children are not aware of the chemical contents of foods or how diet connects to their kidney disorder. Third, younger children tend to be habitual eaters and consume a very limited variety of foods daily. Hence, they not only resist such alterations but by imposing such restrictions one may further limit their overall sources of nutrition and unintentionally promote malnutrition. Fourth, even older children and teenagers find it difficult to comply with dietary restrictions particularly while at school or when visiting friends. They are also reluctant to do so because it may attract attention rather than conceal the fact that they have a kidney disorder. Fifth, swallowing or chewing large pills is a difficult task for nearly all children as well as many adults. Despite these difficulties, a surprisingly large number of my patients paid attention during our clinic encounters when I discussed the rationale for changing their diet. Of course, I congratulated them and their families for their efforts to comply with my recommendations and gave them positive feedback by reviewing improvements in their laboratory data and serial X-ray images.

One of my patients- a ten-year-old boy- presented me with the following amazing cartoon and remarks that indicated a high degree of understanding on his part of the purpose of dietary restrictions. To complement this cartoon and reinforce the positive attitude expressed by this child, I added the following story. The combined handout proved effective in encouraging dietary compliance in other children, in good measure because of my patient's cartoon.

MY KIDNEY, MY HERO

by Demetrius Ellis, M.D.

Illustration by my patient, Christopher B.

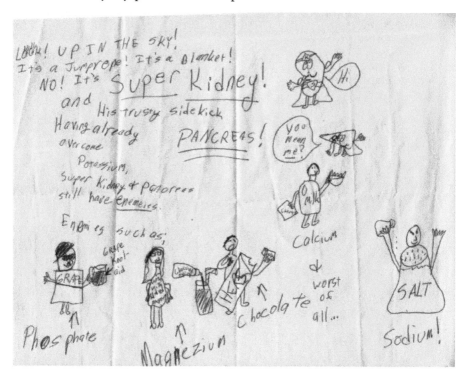

At first, they were loyal friends who respected each other but also guarded their territorial space. They were collectively known as *Molecules*. Their power rested in the knowledge that they were essential in keeping the Body in tip-top condition. Yet they clearly understood that none of them could do this alone; each had a well-defined but limited role and, therefore, had to coexist peacefully with the other Molecules to accomplish this tall order. The Molecules were constantly kept under check by the Body's arch-protector, the Kidney. This was not a simple task because the Body had an appetite for a large range of foods with variable number and kinds of Molecules that only a meticulous, vigilant, and trusted guardian such as the Kidney could regulate. The Molecules were aware of the kidney's priorities and hence,

REFLECTIONS OF "NEPHRON MAN"

if necessary, the Kidney possessed the power to eliminate them as to always maintain this balance. Yet they respected the Kidney not because it was their powerful boss, but because the Kidney was always even-handed, respectful, very modest, and never mistreated them. Therefore, the Molecules behaved well and easily passed the Kidney's inspection when they met with it several times each hour as they circulated via the bloodstream. Of course, Molecules tended to be envious of the Kidney's power and authority, and like children that at times can be mischievous and unruly, they also attempted to test their boundaries. However, their small conspiracies and revolts were no match for the Kidney, and each time, these were quickly squelched in a manner that a kind and loving parent might use to teach a valuable lesson to a child. The Body was grateful for the peace of mind and smooth function of all its organs and had great praise and respect for its appointed taskmaster and guardian, the Kidney.

Then came the unthinkable. Through no fault of its own, the Kidney fell ill. Soon after, its powers began to fade. For the first time in their existence, the Molecules were poorly supervised and free to roam around as the pleased without fear of punishment. They then began to compete with each other and misuse their power. They lost sight of their main mission and the fact that they could not serve the Body effectively by being egotistical and choosing to work independently. For one, Sodium rose so high as to increase the Body's blood pressure to levels that caused headache and challenged the ability of the heart to pump nutrients and oxygen to all the tissues of the Body. Another Molecule, Potassium, which normally worked in partnership with Sodium, Magnesium, and Calcium to maintain the Body's electrical grid, or nervous system, also revolted. As Potassium reached critical levels, the Body feared losing control of all its functions. Another Molecule that typically maintained a low profile in the past, Phosphorus, suddenly became boisterous and a powerful adversary. It demanded greater attention, respect, and acknowledgment of its vital contribution to bone health. In fact, if these demands were not met,

Phosphorus now threatened to inflict bone pain, thereby not allowing playing, running and other physical activities.

Being acutely aware of the Kidney's failing health, Dr. Ellis and his Renal Team had warned the Body of the consequences of the revolt of the Molecules. In fact, Dr. Ellis had previously instructed the Body to follow several dietary modifications and to take a few relatively well-tolerated medications to help restore order among the Molecules and, thereby, avert a catastrophe. However, these changes seemed difficult to implement, and there was an understandable reluctance of the Body to change its daily routine. However, it was clear that the Body used these excuses to hide the painful truth: The Kidney's powers were fading. Faced with the spreading revolt of the Molecules and more ominous and imminent health issues, the Body contacted Dr. Ellis to urgently rescue the Kidney. Because staying mentally and physically active was of paramount importance, the Body capitulated and promised to accept and implement all recommendations. In doing so, the Body also paid homage and gratitude for the years of loyal and courageous service by it's now failing hero, the Kidney.

WELCOME HOME DEMETRI! ATHENS OR BROOKLYN? BOTH!

As a modestly accomplished nephrologist, I was flattered to receive lecture invitations in Athens, Greece where my early education took root, as well as from my chosen homeland, Brooklyn, New York, U.S.A. where I grew up. In Athens, I delivered lectures on pediatric hypertension and urinary tract infections to over seven thousand pediatricians attending the International Pediatric Association Congress in August 2007. I was hosted by the highly accomplished and respected Dr. Constantinos (Dinos) J. Stefanidis and was honored by the Greek Pediatric Nephrology Society that he led.

On another memorable occasion, I was invited to give a lecture in Brooklyn on November 23, 1990, on pediatric renal transplantation. This event was hosted by my aunt, Dr. Stavroula Angelakos-Gabriel— my role model I referred to earlier in the book, and the purpose was to raise funds for the Incurable Illness Foundation. An epicurean dinner was generously served at the Golden Ox, a four-star restaurant owned and managed by my brother, Chris Theodorellis.

My aunt's personal trials and tribulations as a parent of a child with neurologic deficit, as well as her strong social conscience and keen sense of family values shaped her clear vision: children are our future and any efforts to improve their health and instill in them ethical and educational values are the best investments that parents can make. Thus, for her, the need to benefit children with incurable illnesses was a calling awaiting fulfilment. Because the socialized medical system in Greece provided minimal support for such children and their families, this dream could only be realized through private funding. Thus, she conceived of and formed a foundation to raise the money needed to build a facility that could serve as a model for managing children with incurable illnesses. She had the courage of her convictions, relentless energy and commitment, and was eloquent and persuasive. With such personal talents and great resolve, she was unstoppable and nearly always realized her goals. The facility was built in her hometown of Sparta, very close to the exact spot called Apothetae, on top of mount Taiyetos, where the ancient Spartans committed infanticide by throwing into the chasm male children with birth defects, as they were judged incapable of becoming strong warriors.

Among the attendees at the event hosted by my aunt were Manolis Tzitzikalakis, who was one of my first employers during my high school years; my high school and New York University soccer coaches, whom I had not seen for well over twenty years; and the first two girls—now women, that introduced the English language to me when I first arrived to the United States from Greece, just before my thirteenth birthday. Also, in attendance were many Greek-born physicians as well as relatives and friends. The evening raised much money. It was truly enjoyable to be among colleagues, relatives, and childhood friends and to reminisce and catch up on happenings over the intervening years. These events featuring me as a "homegrown professor and scientist" were particularly exhilarating and ego boosting for me, as well as being very memorable.

One notable person who sent a donation but could not attend the above homecoming event in Brooklyn was one of my close college friends, Vassilis Haramis, a brilliant student who became a mathematics professor and mechanical engineer. He was one among thirty-three Greek Americans who had perished in the terrorist attack in New York City on September 11, 2001. I recently contacted his wife, who informed me that Vassilis worked on the ninety-eighth floor of one of the Twin Towers. Based on telephone calls, Vassilis was trying to help an older coworker down the narrow emergency staircase where they encountered many of other individuals who could not escape from the sixty-fifth floor; they all had taken the same route to potential salvation. The building collapsed shortly after. The street on which Vassilis lived was renamed "Haramis Way" in his honor. His profile was published in the *New York Times* on October 25, 2001.

MORE TEACHING ANECDOTES

One of the more memorable incidents in the teaching domain of my career occurred in my first year as a staff member at CHP.

Dr. George Schreiner was the chief of nephrology at Georgetown University in Washington, D.C. He was a renowned researcher and had been elected president of the American Society of Nephrology. He was invited to Pittsburgh to update us on the newly discovered, intriguing pathophysiology of a rare inherited disorder known as *Bartter syndrome*. This disorder clinically presents during childhood with symptoms of increased urine production accompanied by a tendency to dehydration, low blood pressure and dizziness, that is compensated through stimulation of thirst and a desire to drink large volumes of fluids, even during the night; growth retardation is another feature. Low blood potassium levels and increased alkalinity of the blood are commonly noted laboratory features. The condition results from a gene mutation leading to a defective sodium pump at the ascending limb of

Henle in kidney nephrons. The ensuing urinary sodium wasting leads to a state of chronic *hypovolemia* (low blood volume), which triggers secretion of the hormone renin and corresponding hypertrophy of the juxtaglomerular (J-G) apparatus evident on microscopic examination of kidney tissue. In turn, both high renin levels and low blood volume stimulate secretion of aldosterone, a hormone mainly produced by the adrenal glands that stimulates sodium retention, thereby helping to mitigate the symptoms of Bartter syndrome; in the process, aldosterone also reduces blood potassium levels that tend to render the blood more alkaline. These elegant correlations reported by Dr. Schreiner and colleagues provided much insight into normal and aberrant renal physiology, the clinical relevance of which extended well beyond the understanding of Bartter syndrome.

Although Dr. Schreiner came to Pittsburgh at the invitation of my colleagues in adult nephrology, it was suggested that because this was a pediatric topic, I should be the one to introduce him, and I readily agreed. In preparation for this, I would simply look up and briefly summarize Dr. Schreiner's major accomplishments, and then mention the title of his lecture. However, I was overwhelmed by Dr. Schreiner's imposing stature, and after presenting his academic credentials and the topic, I panicked and could not remember his name. At that moment, I turned to the speaker, and with a smile and no hesitation, I pointed to him and said, "And now I present to you a man who needs no introduction."

On another occasion several years later, I stopped for a bathroom break just outside the auditorium where I was to deliver a lecture to the medical students and house staff of CHP. While washing my hands, I noticed that a young man wearing a white jacket typically required of medical students at that time was about to leave the bathroom after urinating without washing his hands. I turned to him and said, "Don't they teach you in medical school to wash your hands after urinating?" He had no idea who I was—he gave me a look that said, *Mind your business* but instead he replied, "No, they teach us not to urinate on our hands."

Shortly after, I entered the auditorium and as I stood at the podium, I instantly made eye contact with the same student who now bit his lip and grinned with embarrassment. To break the ice with this student and to put at ease the rest of the audience, I decided to make a joke out of this bathroom encounter. In a poor imitation of Rodney Dangerfield, I modified one of the favorite lines of the famous comedian and said, "It's not easy being me—I am the Rodney Dangerfield of the nephrology profession. I don't get no respect from medical students or house staff." Without identifying the student who had not washed his hands, I then repeated our ensuing dialogue. However, what I thought was an amusing opening to my lecture, received a lukewarm response. I then realized that I was talking to a younger generation of students, many of whom had no idea of who Rodney Dangerfield was. In similar future encounters I made it a point to consider the age and social and cultural experience-base of my audience, and subsequently had greater success in getting the intended response.

Over the years of my medical practice, I made a conscious effort to find humor even under tragic circumstances. On one occasion early in my career, I was breaking bad news to a young couple whose newborn baby had microcephaly—small head—and neurologic deficit, in addition to a serious renal disorder. I was in the process of explaining that their baby was very likely to be permanently intellectually impaired, when the mother interrupted me and said, "Dr. Ellis, I understand that my baby cannot become a doctor, but can she become a nurse?"

I then realized that either I had not clearly communicated the seriousness of the baby's condition, or the mother was in denial. I hesitated for a moment, and because I could not see any purpose in taking away hope and given the plasticity of the newborn tissues that makes the ultimate neurologic prognosis more difficult to predict with great accuracy, I answered, "Perhaps." Upon hearing this highly unrealistic outlook, the young nurse present in the room could hardly restrain herself from bursting out in laughter. After this incident, I became more reserved in giving outlandish prognoses. Unless I was convinced based on objective clinical criteria that renal (or brain) function was likely to improve, giving false hope for high expectations was not only setting me up for possible litigation but, more importantly, exposed families to much disappointment if the child's condition did not improve in the future.

Research

My personal research and extensive literature review have provided me with insight into the kidney's elegant physiology, pathology, and pathophysiology. Indeed, I openly express my appreciation and extoll the virtues of the kidney in several portions of this book. In fact, this serves as substantial background of much of my *"Advice to my residents and fellows..."* (see, p. 209). Perhaps more so than with other organs systems, renal research has led to a better understanding of the underlying mechanisms of disease processes and has enabled the development of increasingly effective treatment regimens. Although a strong desire to conduct research and a willingness to devote much time and effort into a project are necessary ingredients for success, these attributes are not sufficient to guarantee discovery of meaningful or useful results. From the outset of my career, I had to overcome several obstacles that reduced my chances of success in research. Because of the changing trends in academic medicine, many of the obstacles I faced do not apply to modern-day investigators or physician scientists (see *"What is academic medicine?"*). However, I believe that some of the lessons learned are still pertinent and the application of the tools that I developed to maximize my odds of success may be worthy of consideration by anyone pursuing research in any field of study.

Attaining research tools: Formal instruction in research and laboratory skills is currently mandatory for nearly all new nephrology fellow recruits in the United States. Practical lectures given by experts from various disciplines cover all essential aspects from conceiving a hypothesis, to designing a study, conducting experiments, analyzing data, and publishing results. Bioethics, biostatistics, and grant writing skills are also taught. However, when I began my career, many nephrologists employed in academic centers lacked any such formal instruction or foundation in research. The research skills I developed I owe to my strong commitment and determination to achieve my research goals, as well as to my great fortune of interacting with individuals who helped me acquire them. Thus, a good foundation in the principles of research, coupled with advice and support from an inspiring mentor, can be invaluable.

Be patient! Success takes time: After several years of doing research, I have come to realize that it rarely yields major breakthroughs or eureka moments. It is a slow, arduous, methodical, step-by-step process in which the odds of proving a hypothesis correct, or "rejecting the null hypothesis," are against the scientist. Perhaps these same considerations can also explain why the effort of proving one's hypothesis correct is so rewarding.

Research funding: Although my starting salary at CHP was miniscule, I did manage to negotiate laboratory space and the small sum of $15,000 in start-up funds for research. These resources were grossly inadequate. By maintaining strong collegial relationships with personnel in the neighboring labs, I was able to borrow or barter small amounts of supplies and use some of their technical equipment. Also, I purchased some of my lab supplies through CHP, meaning that I bought certain materials in bulk and at a negotiated institutional discount rate. These maneuvers enabled me to get the most value out of my meager start-up funds.

Protected time for research: Lack of time to devote to research was the biggest impediment to my chances for success. Without devoting sufficient time, meaningful research is not possible. As I indicated previously, my clinical responsibilities were extensive, time-consuming, and unpredictable but constituted my unassailable priority. In addition, as the director of the renal division, I had specific administrative and academic responsibilities that I could not delegate or pass on to other members of my staff or assistants. On aggregate, these unavoidable activities consumed about nine hours of the day, typically from 7:00 a.m. to 4:00 p.m. This left me with roughly four to six hours for research, typically from 4:00 p.m. to 10:00 p.m. After making patient rounds on weekends, I also found time to work in the lab. This was my routine eighty- to ninety-hour weekly schedule at the start of my career. Three years later, when I was able to share clinical responsibilities with Dr. Ellis D. Avner (see "*To give or not to give the mike to EDA?*"), this decreased to about seventy hours per week, so I could devote more time to research. Thus, time constraints were severe during the first three years of my career yet, during that time and against all odds, I managed to complete and publish some exciting and, in my opinion, valuable research projects (see below). What made this possible?

First, as noted above, prolonging my work hours was inevitable. However, this did not seem such a harsh sacrifice because I really enjoyed what I was doing. I speculated that as my renal staff grew in number, I would eventually have the prospect of more personal and family time. In addition, I reasoned that, if I succeeded in obtaining promising preliminary data, I could apply for financial support from outside grant agencies and thus pursue more ambitious investigations in the future. These funds could enable me to hire lab techs who could do much of the daily work under minimal supervision. However, I was keenly aware that such strategy would not save me as much time as it seemed because my physical presence was needed to set up and conduct the initial lab experiments, resolve routine problems encountered in the lab each day, and oversee the work of the lab techs to ensure the results' validity and avoid fabrication. I firmly believe that an absentee investigator cannot succeed in research. In any case, developing an optimistic long-term outlook of my future strengthened my resolve to focus on making progress each day.

Second, I declined certain departmental tasks and some administrative meetings that I considered nonessential for managing the renal division. I also avoided volunteering for some hospital and university committees. My only de facto boss, the chairman of pediatrics, as well as the other division chiefs at CHP were aware of the long hours I devoted to my patients and the expert and expeditious consults I provided to patients on the wards. My teaching contributions were also extensive and well received. Thus, all my colleagues were aware that I was not slacking off, and no one ever gave me the impression that my actions placed an extra burden on them.

Third, because of success with my systematic approach to improving my efficiency while performing my clinical duties (see "*Demetri, a model of efficiency*"), I also tried to become creative with maximizing my use of time in conducting research. To accomplish this, I chose to investigate highly selected hypotheses and projects that were not only interesting and relevant to patient care but would also increase my motivation and effort to carry them to their successful completion. This required more work on my part up front, in the preplanning stages. This project preselection and logistical process, together with focusing on only one or two projects at any one time and making wise use of my time, were invaluable for my research success. In addition, an element of luck along the way was most welcome.

OVERVIEW OF SELECTED
LABORATORY PROJECTS AND CLINICAL STUDIES

Among my laboratory projects was the development of a unique approach for isolating one renal cell type, proximal tubular epithelial cells, from mouse kidneys using a novel magnetic/antibody technique. I then ascertained that these *primary cells* maintained their specialized function after I succeeded in growing them in culture media. Once the cells multiplied and covered the entire plate, I used them to investigate corticosteroid receptors. Although other investigators purchased readily available immortalized cell lines to conduct similar experiments, the primary or freshly prepared cells that I painstakingly extracted and used in my work provided more physiologically pertinent results. In fact, my experiments provided insight into how renal cells respond to steroids that are commonly administered orally or intravenously to manage several human disorders. I then used a variation of this technique to grow primary human tubular epithelial cells in hollow fibers encased in an ordinary dialyzer in an attempt to develop a primitive artificial kidney. Presently, there is a resurgence of interest in developing such a kidney.

In contrast to my basic or laboratory-based research, compared to other nephrologists, my clinical research interests tended to be broad, rather than focused, reflecting my fascination with the multiple intricate renal functions; after all, the kidney is the *quintessence of form-structure and function*" (see p. 121). I describe a few of these clinical projects below.

Because of my scientific contributions, I was granted membership to the very selective and prestigious Society of Pediatric Research. In addition, I was an active member in the American Academy of Pediatrics and served as an editor of *Pediatric Nephrology* and several other pediatric and adult nephrology journals. Unfortunately, because of the unanticipated relocation of some of my clinical staff, I faced intermittent workforce shortages, forcing me to double up on my clinical responsibilities. This resulted in lengthy interruptions in my basic research efforts, such that it became increasingly difficult to maintain an active research lab. Consequently, for the last twenty years of my career, I pursued clinical research exclusively.

My involvement in research availed me many memorable, exciting, interesting, and amusing, if not instructive, experiences that I would never have had if I had pursued a private or nonacademic practice of medicine. I believe that several of the anecdotes that follow provide the reader with unique glimpses of my research experience.

DR. DAVID G

A very accomplished and world renown pediatric immunologist, Dr. David G, had previously used the lab that I inherited at CHP. He had devised his own electrophoresis and invented several other apparatuses that helped him pioneer research on maternal-to-fetus antibody transfer across the placenta. He had also conducted extensive research on viruses, vaccines, and antibody responses in children. Dr. G stored much of the equipment and chemical supplies that he used in a closet in the hallway of the original CHP facility. In fact, this closet contained many of the supplies and reagents that I needed for my own experiments.

About six months after working in my lab, I and all others involved in research received a notice from an administrator requesting us to conduct an inventory of our equipment and supplies. By identifying which of these were purchased and used individually by multiple researchers, CHP could use its purchasing power to ultimately realize substantial savings by buying these in bulk. Special sheets were provided for tabulating this information. In the process of going through the materials in the closet one afternoon, I became instantly petrified and had goose bumps as I read the label on the dark-blue jar that I was holding: "smallpox." I washed my hands vigorously and several times after handling this vial. Fortunately, I did not open it. I then immediately contacted Dr. Richard Michaels, our infectious disease chief, who, in turn, contacted the Center for Disease Control (CDC) and Prevention in Atlanta, Georgia. Within a few minutes, we received a call from the CDC instructing us to cordon off the area immediately and to require everyone on that hospital floor to remain in place. We were informed that a team equipped to handle such an *emergency* was preparing to be dispatched from the CDC. Indeed, within a few hours, several people dressed in Hazmat suits arrived to remove and neutralize what apparently was live and deadly smallpox virus. Since then, the CDC has formulated multiple safety measures to guard against potentially lethal environmental disasters related to research utilizing infectious agents.

HIEN

Another memorable incident involved one my laboratory technicians, Hien. This woman had left South Vietnam after the end of the Vietnam War in 1975. She had a thick but pleasant French-Vietnamese accent blend and pronounced her broken English in a very low tone. Her main lab expertise was in maintaining cell cultures; she did a commendable job in separating and growing the particularly intricate fresh kidney cells described above. I quickly learned that Hien went out of her way to avoid all social and professional interaction with the other lab techs on that floor. Instead, she preferred to work independently. She did not befriend, ask for help, or exchange any supplies from any other of the more sociable techs working in proximity to our lab. When I asked her to explain her behavior, she would say, "I am scared they sabotage our work." She also exhibited several other signs of mistrust bordering on paranoid behavior. Hien volunteered very little personal information, but I suspected she had experienced mental or emotional trauma during the Vietnam War.

At one point, our experiments required the use of low-level radioactive labeling. One day while Hien was routinely monitoring for radioactivity in our sterile hood, the Geiger counter detected what seemed to be a high amount of radioactivity. Hien immediately became alarmed and paged me over the public announcement system of the hospital. When I called her, speaking quickly in an agitated manner and with a thicker accent than usual, she conveyed to me that she was concerned because "exposure to high radioactivity harm my baby." This surprised me because I was not aware that she was pregnant and, although I did not know her precise age, she appeared to be in her late forties and, presumably, beyond child-bearing age. I asked her to calm down and assured her that we had not purchased any reagents with the high level of radiation she had detected. I also assured her that I was coming to the lab immediately to investigate her concerns. I arrived at our lab a few minutes later and encountered several lab personnel congregating outside the women's bathroom/locker room located across from our lab. They informed me that Hien had locked herself in the bathroom and refused to open the door. Speaking through the closed door, I again tried to convince her that the radioactivity level she had detected was of minimal danger to her, but she was skeptical and insisted that I did not have sufficient expertise to make this prediction. I agreed with her and explained that I would consult several experts from other departments at the University of Pittsburgh. In the meantime, I expressed great concern about her well-being and implored her to come out of the bathroom, so she could get some lunch and meet personally with the experts. However, she remained locked-up. This did not permit the other techs to gain access to their purses, keys and other belongings when it was time for them to go home.

During that time, a physics professor, a biochemist, and a gynecologist/obstetrician with special expertise in infant/mother complications related to environmental exposures, including radiation, all came to assuage Hien. In the meantime, we discovered that the radiation was actually emanating from across the corner wall of the adjacent clinical lab and not from our own research hood. It took the experts and me about six hours to persuade Hien to finally open the door. About 14 months later, Hien had a healthy daughter who is currently about thirty years old.

Although Hien stopped working for me three decades ago, she still visits me every Christmas and brings me a bottle of whiskey. For reasons unknown to me, she has changed employment on multiple occasions. She still refers to me as "boss" and requests that I serve as a work reference for her. Of course, my comments relating to her professional competence and work ethic are always complimentary.

RESEARCH GONE AWRY

In 1993, our older daughter, Melissa, graduated from Princeton University and matriculated at medical school. I am convinced that this milestone had its genesis in infancy. When she was barely two years old, my wife and Melissa visited me regularly while I was a resident at CHP and had thirty-six-hour shifts every three days. Their evening visits allowed us to dine on Irene's exceptional cooking and to spend quality time together. One evening, Melissa stopped by the human-ized bronze statue of Fred, a life-size bear, complete with a hat, located in the lobby at CHP. She gave Fred lollipops and with a great deal of conviction said, "When I grow up, I will become a physician, just like my dad."

Because showing a strong interest in science was desirable when applying to medical schools, in 1992, Melissa and her cousin Michael, who was also applying to med school, requested to work in my lab. Their main task was to maintain the precious cell cultures that I used in experiments related to diabetic kidney disease. I was in need of lab techs then and I also thought that it would be a great opportunity for both Melissa and Michael to interact socially; so, I hired them. Despite my best efforts to educate this dynamic duo on the importance of sterile technique, all my cultures became contaminated and quickly died. Upon completing medical school, neither of them pursued basic research, but both are currently gifted physicians and serve as fine role models.

Four years after this lab incident and unknown to me at the time, when applying to pediatric residency programs, Melissa was interviewed by a preeminent pediatric nephrologist at the Cleveland Clinic—Dr. Robert Cunningham. Several years afterwards, I was invited to lec-ture there on pediatric transplantation. In his introduction of me, Dr. Cunningham informed the audience and me that he had interviewed my daughter several years earlier and said that he remembered her well partly because of her unique answers to his questions. He recalled for the audience that when he asked Melissa why she chose to pursue a pediatric career, she replied, "When I was growing up, I was influenced by a god masquerading as my father." This was the most magnanimous compliment I'd ever received. Of course, I must admit that although

Melissa has always been bright and articulate, in this instance, she may have slightly exaggerated my prowess. Melissa went on to become a splendid pediatrician. Her longitudinal and comprehensive program benefiting homeless children and families in the Philadelphia, PA area is highly effective and meritorious.

One of the proudest moments of my career was just prior to Melissa's graduation from medical school and just before the start of her residency program at the Children's Hospital of Philadelphia. She elected to come to CHP to do a one-month pediatric nephrology elective with me, as well as a cardiology elective. Her cardiology attending was a highly respected former Harvard trainee—Dr. Fred Sherman—whom I knew well. However, he did not realize that Melissa was my daughter until the very last day of her cardiology elective. He then informed me that he had never met any student or trainee that was as thorough and efficient in extracting clinically relevant information, particularly from teenagers who tend to be secretive and guarded in divulging details about their personal habits. He was very impressed and complimentary of her. During those two months, her identification tag read, Melissa Ellis, M.D. I recall how proud I was as we walked the hallways of CHP together and I introduced her to my patients as "my daughter, the other Dr. Ellis". A month later, her identification tag read, "Melissa Ellis Bennett, M.D.," reflecting her recent marriage.

I would be remiss if I did not say a few words about our younger daughter, Trish. She chose a nonmedical career. As a talented urban planner, she and her team have the monumental and unenviable task of keeping public transportation up and running smoothly daily in the city of Philadelphia, PA. As with her sister, Trish's innovative ideas and dedication to her work also serve the people of that fine city.

Diabetes and the fabulous "Nephelometer"

During a large portion of my career, I was most privileged to be part of an outstanding, dedicated, and productive team investigating renal and other complications related to diabetes mellitus. The story that follows describes how I came to be a member of this group and is a great example of how progress in seemingly unrelated medical fields, such as nephrology and endocrinology, converge to advance medical knowledge.

Diabetes mellitus is a serious disorder at any age. The childhood variety is known as *type I diabetes* (T1D) or insulin-dependent diabetes. This is a virulent form of diabetes in which the pancreas's insulin production is deficient. Proper management includes blood sugar testing several times daily and adjustments to the multiple daily insulin injections. This contrasts with the adult form that is often associated with obesity—also known as *type II diabetes* (T2D)— that is typically managed with oral medications and dietary approaches. The medical complications of both forms are equally serious but occur in a much shorter period after the onset of T1D. One of the more devastating complications is renal failure requiring dialysis or kidney transplantation; concomitant pancreas transplantation may also cure the diabetes. Why certain people develop kidney failure while others do not is not entirely clear, although poor long-term blood sugar control is a major contributor.

In the late 1970s, epidemiologic studies showed that individuals with T1D who exhibited small but higher than normal albumin excretion in their urine—or microalbuminuria—had a much higher chance of developing renal failure during the succeeding decade. Several subsequent studies indicated that the microalbuminuria could be reversed, and the renal failure delayed or prevented through intensive blood glucose control over time. Thus, early detection of microalbumin excretion offered the prospect of markedly reducing the chances of developing diabetic nephropathy. However, this low level of albumin excretion noted in the very early stages of renal disease is too small to be detected by the typical urine dipsticks available at most doctors' offices. Moreover, only a few research laboratories could measure such low urinary albumin levels, while nearly all hospital laboratories lacked a precise, clinically applicable method of doing so.

Pediatrics focuses on preventive aspects of disease perhaps more than any other medical specialty. The best example of this is the world-wide use of immunizations. Thus, discovering a practical method for early detection of renal disease and the implied greater therapeutic benefit through potential earlier interventions was very appealing to me. As I noted earlier in the book, this notion had motivated me during my fellowship in Washington, D.C. to collaborate with Gregory Buffone, Ph.D., to develop a nephelometric method for detection of subclinical levels of urinary albumin. This was a technically tedious method in which a sample of the patient's urine was reacted in a test tube containing a special solution containing a commercially available antibody to human albumin. The more albumin contained in the sample, the more cloudy the fluid became. The degree of cloudiness, or *nephelos*, from the Greek word for "cloud," was then quantified using an analog meter or a needle, like the familiar voltage detector, the movement of which corresponded to the amount of light scattered by the albumin-antibody complexes. The value was then compared to a standard curve generated by using known amounts of purified human albumin available commercially and incubated with antibody in an identical manner as the patient samples. The method proved to be relatively simple, more sensitive in detecting tiny amounts of albumin, and more reproducible and precise than previous methods, thus making it more suitable for general laboratory use. The biggest drawback of this method was eyestrain related to reading the very sensitive and often unstable analog meter needle. The solution to this dilemma was better equipment. When a medical equipment manufacturer —Hyland Co.—learned of this problem, they made available to me an engineer from their instrument development unit. After spending considerable time with me in my lab and becoming familiar with the existing method, this ingenious individual went to work. His team then engineered a prototype of the Hyland nephelometer, complete with an early application of the then-budding laser technology as the light source and a much-welcome digital, rather than analog, readout. After several modifications, we reported the clear advantages, including sensitivity and specificity, of our method compared to preexisting methods (A new approach to the evaluation of proteinuric states. Clin Chem 23:666, 1977). Upon my graduation from fellowship, Hyland Co. presented me with the prototype, which I took with me to Pittsburgh. At that time, it was valued at about $50,000, or about 1.5 times my annual salary.

Soon after its publication, our method was in great demand because of the contemporaneous and fortuitous publication of the above-noted studies indicating the clinical significance of microalbuminuria as a harbinger of diabetic renal disease. I received multiple offers to participate in studies involving individuals with T1D. In fact, I and my lab were contracted to serve as the central lab for measuring urinary albumin and other measures of kidney function in a large multicenter trial conducted by the pharmaceutical manufacturer, Pfizer Inc., involving management of diabetic polyneuropathy with an aldose reductase inhibitor named Sorbinil (The sorbinil retinopathy trial: neuropathy results. Sorbinil Retinopathy Trial Research Group. Neurology 43:1141-1149, 1993). Incidentally, this study was done in the late 1970s and did not show significant benefit; however, currently there has been a resurgence of interest in using a similar agent based on preliminary studies demonstrating much greater effectiveness when this is used starting at an earlier phase of diabetic polyneuropathy. The funds received for my performance of microalbuminuria and assessment of renal function were significant and together with those obtained from other sources, supported my research lab for many years after completion of this study.

This background explains how as a young pediatric nephrologist, I was invited to participate in the very important investigation alluded to in the introduction of this section. Under the exceptional leadership of Dr. Trevor Orchard, we received approval and funding from the National Institutes of Health to study the natural history and multiple complications in 657 adults in the Pittsburgh and Western Pennsylvania area diagnosed with TID at an average age of about ten. As you might guess, I was primarily responsible for assessing the renal complications of individuals enrolled in this large population-based study. My tasks consisted of measuring albumin levels in serum and urine, as well as evaluating overall renal function in these individuals. The employment of the original technique to measure microalbuminuria throughout the duration of this longitudinal study has provided unparalleled uniformity of results. Indeed, this study is currently in its twenty-fifth year and is highly cited by many experts in the field because it has identified several important factors that can be modified as to prevent or ameliorate the progression of renal disease and other catastrophic complications. Key publications include: Choice of urine samples predictive of microalbuminuria in patients with insulin-dependent diabetes mellitus. Am J Kidney Dis 13:321-328, 1989; The detection of microalbuminuria in insulin-dependent diabetes mellitus: An assessment of AlbuSure, a screening tests. Diabetes Care 12:389-393, 1989; Diabetes complications and glycemic control. The Pittsburgh Prospective Insulin-Dependent Diabetes Cohort Study (PPIDDCo): status report after 5 years of IDDM. Diabetes Care 12:694-700, 1989; Factors associated with avoidance of severe complications after 25 years of IDDM. Pittsburgh Epidemiology of Diabetes Complications Study II. Diabetes Care 13:741-747, 1990; Predictors of microalbuminuria in individuals with IDDM. Pittsburgh Epidemiology of diabetes complications study. Diabetes Care 16(10)1376-1383, 1993; The changing course of diabetes nephropathy: LDL-cholesterol and blood pressure correlate with regression of proteinuria. Am J Kidney Dis 27(6):809-818, 1996; Sequence of progression of albuminuria and decreased GFR in persons with type 1 diabetes: a cohort study. Am J Kidney Dis 2007; 50(5):721-732; Changing impact of modifiable risk factors on the incidence of major outcomes of Type 1 diabetes. The Pittsburgh Epidemiology of Diabetes Complications Study. Diabetes Care care.diabetesjournals.org. Epidemiology/Health Services Research. Diabetes Care, Publications Ahead of Print, published online October 29, 2013; Urinary microRNA profiling in the nephropathy of type 1 diabetes. J Clin Med. 2015 Jul; 4(7): 1498–1517.

I never could have envisioned how my relatively simple technique and the nephelometer would eventually fetch me so much fortune and fame. It was as though I had won the jackpot. Although its best days are over, my nephelometer is still functioning after forty-one years. A picture of me and my prized nephelometer is shown below.

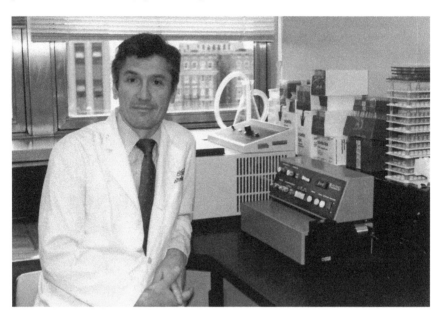

Because microalbuminuria is still considered an important marker of renal and other microvascular complications of diabetes, it is monitored on a routine basis. Testing is available in nearly all clinical and hospital laboratories in the United States. An automated version of our original nephelometric technique remains a preferred method.

WATER INTOXICATION IN INFANTS

An interesting but mysterious disorder that I helped unravel is the development of new-onset seizures in otherwise healthy infants with no apparent head injury or other provocation. The cause was water intoxication. Babies with this disorder presented with seizures occurring between four and eight months of age, and *hyponatremia*, reduced blood levels of sodium; both the hyponatremia and seizures resolved after a spontaneous increase in urine production during a period of eight to twelve hours after admission. The mothers were usually inexperienced first-time mothers who seemed to be especially anxious and stressed when faced with caring for their infant and tended to allow their babies to drink water, sometimes to the exclusion of milk and baby foods. In short, I had suspected a psycho-behavioral cause leading to a preference for water over milk or baby food intake. The underlying mechanism of the apparent water intoxication was not readily evident, but previous experience indicated that it did not take much water retention to cause the seizures. This condition is rare among healthy infants because the normal body response is to decrease or suppress secretion of antidiuretic hormone (ADH), resulting in a spontaneous increase in sodium-free urine production, thereby guarding against reduction of blood sodium concentration. Therefore, I hypothesized that in infants with water intoxication, "an aberrant or high secretion of ADH impaired the ability of the kidneys to excrete a water load." However, owing to the fleeting nature of this condition, one must measure ADH concentrations immediately upon arrival in the Emergency Department (ED). In addition, brain trauma and other more common conditions that cause a similar electrolyte imbalance and symptoms had to be excluded. Because it was not possible for me to be physically present in the ED at all hours, I elicited the help of a most capable senior resident, Dr. Ron David. He had previously taken care of an infant with this condition while on a month-long renal elective with me and was interested in helping me document future cases. Dr. David alerted the ED staff to contact him personally, so he could explain the protocol that we jointly devised to identify and study these babies expeditiously. Over the next six months, we encountered two infants with this condition. We measured plasma ADH and performed renal and urine studies on initial presentation, as well as after eight hours of withholding all water intake. Urine studies and urine output as well as free water clearance were also measured simultaneously. To our great satisfaction, the time course of clinical improvement correlated well with normalization in ADH and blood sodium levels. The rapid reversal of this disorder tended to exclude a structural brain disorder or kidney malfunction. Rather, our data supported our suspicion that the mother's anxiety and stress of caring for their infant transferred to the baby. The concurrent offering of water by the mother may have reinforced the infant's water-drinking habit and perhaps stimulated hunger and further stress that are recognized triggers of ADH secretion. With this somewhat theoretical or presumed scenario of the initiating events, the objective corroborative laboratory measurements, and favorable clinical response in these infants, we provided the mothers with counselling aimed at preventing recurrences of the disorder. Indeed, the infants remained well on follow-up monitoring. Subsequently, we succeeded in publishing our study in a very reputable journal (David R and Ellis D: Water intoxication in normal infants. Role of antidiuretic hormone. *Pediatrics* 69:349, 1981).

More than three decades later, Dr. Ron David gave an update on this disorder at a pediatric grand rounds lecture at DuPont Hospital. This presentation was given in honor of the retirement of a mutual, highly respected colleague, Dr. Carl Gardner. Dr. David did a scholarly literature review of this topic and uncovered several recent articles in which various hypotheses were proposed to explain the condition. He concluded that our original hypothesis and laboratory data provided the most convincing explanation. This is consistent with one of the basic tenets in medicine—Occam's razor, (Latinized name of 14th century theologian and philosopher, William of Ockham), or *the law of parsimony*. According to this principle, a hypothesis that makes the fewest assumptions and largely explains the observed findings is the most easily tested and the most likely to prove correct. Throughout my career, I have made a concerted effort to apply this minimalist approach to the diagnosis of medical conditions (see p. 218). However, one should be acutely aware that when confronted with a medical emergency, over analysis can lead to indecision and delays of needed interventions with potentially disastrous consequences.

Systemic lupus erythematosus (SLE)

Another condition of great interest to me is systemic lupus erythematosus (SLE). It is an autoimmune disorder with a familial and female predilection. Because of diffuse inflammation of small vessels, or *vasculitis*, SLE can affect all organs in the body and is therefore known as the "great masquerader," much as syphilis was in the past. The disorder predominantly affects the skin, joints, as well as the kidney (*lupus nephritis* or *SLE glomerulonephritis*). Thus, most patients with SLE are managed by rheumatologists and referred to nephrologists when needed. SLE occurs less frequently in children than in adults, and lupus nephritis is even less likely to have an onset in childhood. During my nephrology fellowship in Washington, D.C., I had personal experience with five severely affected adolescents with this disorder. Their outlook was dismal.

On arrival at CHP, there was no service dedicated to pediatric rheumatology and very few children with SLE were admitted to CHP, but within days of my arrival, I encountered my first patient with lupus nephritis. The renal aspects were completely overshadowed by the orthopedic issues in this unfortunate sixteen-year-old African American male. AD had severe arthritis and had received a large cumulative amount of prednisone to suppress the inflammation. The steroid's side effects were striking. He had marked Cushingoid appearance with a round or moon face, diabetes, thin arms and legs with muscle atrophy and proximal muscle weakness, truncal obesity with protuberant abdomen, and compression fractures of several lumbar and thoracic vertebrae. He also suffered from headaches related to systemic hypertension as well as *pseudotumor cerebri* (swelling of the optic nerves) evident upon examining the posterior part of the eyes. AD's outdoor activities consisted exclusively of bowling. I first met him shortly after a bowling outing; because of severe osteoporosis, even this low amount of physical stress had caused yet another vertebra fracture requiring admission to CHP. The resulting back pain was excruciating and proved difficult to manage. He also had decreased urine output which together with a newly increased serum creatinine level indicated an acute reduction in kidney function. There were no abnormal amounts of protein or blood in the urine to suggest severe glomerular or vascular disease related to lupus nephritis. To exclude pain from kidney stones and possible acute blockage of the ureters thereby limiting urine flow from the kidneys to the bladder, I obtained an *intravenous pyelogram* (a commonly performed test at that time in which X-rays are obtained after an injection of a liquid in a vein that is concentrated in the kidneys and excreted in the urine). I was in disbelief at finding severe, almost 180-degree, malrotation or twisting of his kidneys, and partial ureteral obstruction. This was caused by several golf-ball-sized balls of fat around the kidneys. Extensive literature search disclosed a single similar case. I have never encountered this condition since then.

Despite all these complications, AD was upbeat. Eventually, he developed extensive complications mainly related to steroid use and died within a year. Clearly, the treatment was worse than the disease for this young man.

Over the ensuing years, I encountered many adolescents with SLE. Before an amazing rheumatologist, Dr. Vincent "Vinny" Landino, joined our staff, I was often their main caretaker. During my career, I performed kidney biopsies on well over a hundred of these children, and I was frequently appalled by the degree of renal inflammation and features suggestive of rapid progression of the disease within days of their initial clinical presentation. Clearly, these findings called for urgent and intensive management. At that time, treatment typically consisted of prolonged use of high-dose oral steroids and cyclophosphamide. This approach was not associated with prolonged remission, while major side effects were common, including sterility related to cyclophosphamide (a well-known side effect of this widely utilized chemotherapeutic agent). Steroid toxicity, though not as severe as in AD, was also universally present. Thus, a more effective treatment regimen was urgently needed.

In late 1979, Dr. Anthony Fauci at the National Institutes of Health presented promising preliminary results in adults with severe lupus nephritis managed with a new protocol. This consisted of high-dose intravenous methylprednisolone (IV or pulse steroid therapy) for three days followed by lower daily oral steroid dosages, together with a single monthly intravenous cyclophosphamide injection for six months. This more aggressive initial treatment strategy arrested disease progression more quickly while affording a significant steroid-sparing effect in the long term. Consequently, the efficacy-to-adverse effect ratio markedly improved. I then modified this regimen for use in children and later included harvesting eggs from the ovaries of ovulating females, to permit them to have biological children later in adulthood. This regimen proved of great benefit to my patients. Over the past two decades, I largely replaced cyclophosphamide with a less toxic agent, mycophenolate mofetil or CellCept (F. Hoffman-La Roche AG). This enabled me and other nephrologists to make further progress with curbing steroid use.

OTHER GLOMERULONEPHRITIDES

Besides SLE, there are several other serious acute and chronic disorders that predominantly affect the small vascular tufts of the kidney, or *glomeruli*, whose task is to filter the blood. These disorders are grouped under the heading of *glomerulonephritides*, and some are also suspected of having an autoimmune or immunologic cause. Depending on the severity of injury, an evaluation may disclose a variable degree of urinary protein loss, dark or bloody urine, diffuse body swelling, high blood pressure, renal dysfunction, and the prospect of progressive renal injury leading to permanent renal failure and transplantation. No effective or standardized treatment existed for many of these disorders.

Starting in 1995, I began to manage several glomerulonephritides including severe IgA nephritis, protracted post-infectious glomerulonephritis, certain forms of steroid unresponsive nephrotic syndrome, and other conditions utilizing a two-drug regimen. An agent called losartan (Merck & Company, Inc.) helped lower the protein loss in the urine while concurrently protecting the kidneys against the injurious effect of high blood pressure that can occur within the glomeruli in several glomerulonepritides. CellCept (described above in connection with SLE) was added to reduce the body's immune-mediated damaging effect on glomeruli. As later demonstrated in various animal models of glomerulonephritis, the two agents acted synergistically, which explained the superior clinical response in my patients, while side effects were considerably lower compared to previous treatment regimens. Over the years, this drug combination received much acclaim and is currently used with much success worldwide.

Based on a review of the effectiveness and safety of the use of losartan in over a hundred children managed principally under my supervision, Merck & Company Inc. applied and received approval from the Food and Drug Administration for the use of losartan in children. In addition, I brought attention to the hazards of combining agents belonging to the same class as losartan (angiotensin receptor blockers or ARBs, and agents of a closely related class [ACE inhibitors]), a common practice in the past that is currently avoided.

SCIENTIFIC WRITING

Conceiving a hypothesis, designing, and funding a research study is a very time-consuming process; it takes much effort and determination to carry a study to its successful completion. Once the study is finally completed, it is of limited value unless the findings are disseminated and confirmed independently by other investigators. To this end, one must first determine which scientific journal is most suitable for the subject matter and the intended readership. Certain pediatric journals publish articles on multiple pediatric disciplines, while other journals tend to publish articles that are more suitable to a specific pediatric specialty. One must closely adhere to the directions for the authors, which are often complex and unique to each journal. Regardless of the journal, however, when writing scientific articles, one must always substantiate each important statement by quoting previously published investigations. In such writing, embellishment, humor, or remarks that reflect the author's personality are strictly avoided; one must always adhere to the facts and subject the results to rigorous statistical analysis for the study to be credible and have a chance of publication. Also, unlike prose that may be written expressly for the enjoyment of the reader, the main objective of articles found in medical journals is to add to the understanding of the pathophysiology of a medical disorder. After several edits of an article, the hope is that it will be published and make its way in academia. In the process, one gains a reputation within their specialty while simultaneously garnering prestige for their institution and university. This is also of practical importance when submitting one's curriculum vitae for consideration for academic promotion.

RESEARCH AND PRIVATE GIFTS

Research conducted at many university-associated centers benefits society by fostering the discovery of new technologies and medications that ultimately aid diagnosis and management. Translational research has emerged as a popular model for investigating specific disorders more efficiently and effectively. This involves recruiting individuals with diverse scientific expertise or knowledge such as physiology, genetics, biochemistry, biotechnology, and medicine. Having such teams of experts increases the odds for medical institutions to successfully compete for research funding, from the National Institutes of Health or from several large organizations that raise funds for the study of cancer, diabetes, and specific disorders of the brain, heart, kidney, and other organs. Success in this endeavor enhances the recruitment of more exceptional scientists, resulting in the development of renowned clinical programs that attract even more patients and lead to greater overall growth of these programs. Thus, a strong research program makes good business sense. While large amounts of funding obtained from highly competitive granting sources, such as the National Institutes of Health, bring much prestige and raise an institute's national ranking, other funds raised by local institutions and private donors are also very important. These funds support the construction of new physical facilities, supplement research funding, provide free clinical care to socially and financially disadvantaged individuals, and support programs more directly related to patient care. Although all contributions are accepted, the more generous private donors are often honored by attaching their names to medical buildings or special fund designations.

Over my medical career, I had the privilege and great fortune to interact with several private donors. Whenever I thought appropriate, I informed potential donors that members of my own nephrology division were conducting research on medical conditions that had affected their loved ones. Thus, although I never directly solicited donations for any of our programs, this was tacitly assumed. In addition, upon request from the CHP Development Fund, I did furnish the names of potential donors. These individuals were then invited to attend a formal presentation, typically delivered by the physician in charge of the respective research project. Within a couple days, the donors would be approached to discuss the specific objectives that their intended gift would support. It was in this context that I became personally acquainted with the late Elsie H. Hillman. In 2005, Mr. and Mrs. Hillman made a very generous gift to establish the Hillman Center for Pediatric Transplantation to support research and clinical programs related to transplantation at CHP. To my great satisfaction, the Hillmans as well as other donors had one major condition for donating: "Dr. Demetrius Ellis's nephrology service should benefit from our donation." My admiration and deep appreciation for the kindness and great generosity of both small and large donors cannot be overstated. I am forever grateful for my association with and support from these families.

The following is a handwritten letter from Mrs. Hillman after I gave a research presentation to her and Mr. Hillman. Among the other attendees were the head of CHP Foundation, Mr. Craig; the chairman of pediatrics, Dr. Perlmutter; and the new chief of pediatric nephrology, Carl Bates.

June 16 '10

Dear Greg —
Please accept, on behalf of all your wonderful group, our thanks for a very special day at the Children's Hospital. Every part was perfect for us! Rachel planned a great and delicious luncheon, and the flowers were beautiful, too!) the speakers were each so articulate about their subjects and so gracious to us. We felt very included into their stories and comments and, I hope, us come away "smarter".

Our session with Dr. Ellis, Dr. Baker and Dr. Perlmutter was very special to me. I am anxious to learn more as we move along on the nephrotic syndrome problem.

Please tell Hoddy and all others how grateful we are for their time and their commitment to Children's! Gratefully and best wishes, Elsie H.

PERSONAL RESEARCH CONTRIBUTIONS

One must be cautious in taking personal credit for advancing a scientific field, particularly given today's investigational sophistication and the team effort needed to design and complete a study. Due credit must first be conferred to prior researchers who advanced one or more aspect of investigation. With these caveats, I have personally had a leadership role in conducting studies that substantially contributed to the understanding or management of several disorders and, therefore, share much or part of the credit for the scientific publications bearing my name.

Over my forty-two years in nephrology, children who presented with largely untreatable and progressive renal disorders often fueled my desire to develop innovative interventions. In my opinion, the cliché "necessity is the mother of invention" applies to medicine as much if not more than any other field. A common thread of most of my research contributions is that the research findings are of practical value and have passed the test of time, as many of them have become the standard of care worldwide. My motivation and determination to undertake new approaches emanated directly from the need to resolve challenging medical conditions that threatened the very lives of my patients. My seminal investigations relate to renal transplantation, high blood pressure in children, and diabetic kidney disease.

As I have mentioned previously (p. 93), prior to 1981, transplantation of all organs was hampered because of ineffective immunosuppressive drugs needed to control organ rejection. By mere serendipity, in 1981, I joined a team that pioneered the use of cyclosporine, a modern-era drug that revolutionized organ transplants. Similarly, starting in December 1987, we further advanced this field through the initial use of tacrolimus, an even more effective and safer agent. To this day, tacrolimus-based immunosuppressive protocols continue to be the most popular worldwide. WHat is often forgotten, however, is that determining the effective dosage and limiting side effects of these powerful agents was a challenging endeavor (see pp. 186 and 187). I vividly recall the first child that received tacrolimus after renal transplantation. This ten-year-old girl did well after the transplant, but despite appearing well and fully able to hear and understand my questions, two days later, she could not utter a single word (*expressive aphasia*). This concerning neurologic symptom was initially unexplained until three days later when we received the blood tacrolimus level result from the central Abbott Lab—it was toxic. It turned out that, like cyclosporine, tacrolimus is lipophilic and, therefore, tends to accumulate preferentially in fatty tissues such as the brain, nerves and pancreas, which explains its neurotoxicity and effects on insulin. We immediately lowered her tacrolimus dosage, and her aphasia completely resolved within a few days. She is currently employed as a paralegal. She and other brave children undergoing transplantation under experimental medication protocols enabled us to optimize the drug dosages and define and manage side effects. Therefore, they deserve much of the credit for paving the way for future children to experience better transplant outcomes and higher quality of life.

Tacrolimus use also improved the outlook of children with a most challenging disorder called *focal and segmental glomerulosclerosis*. Most children with this condition present with severe protein loss in the urine, resulting in diffuse body swelling, or *nephrotic syndrome*, and typically show little or no response to steroids or other medications; most children develop severe renal failure within ten years. After initiation of tacrolimus in 1988, over 50% of children achieved full remission while many others had partial remission; only a minority of children developed progressive renal failure.

I was the first to enroll children with intractable high blood pressure in the initial trial of minoxidil, and later on, I was the only pediatric nephrologist consulted in the labetalol trial. Both agents were effective. However, unlike several existing agents that could lower blood pressure, labetalol did not interfere with the metabolism or blood levels of cyclosporine or tacrolimus and did not reduce renal blood flow. Hence, labetalol proved useful in the management of high blood pressure occurring in children with a variety of organ transplants, which was especially common with use of cyclosporine+/- steroids. In additions, Dr. Ron Shapiro, who led our surgical renal transplant team at CHP, and I developed a very successful protocol for bilateral renal auto-transplantation to manage intractable hypertension in children with bilateral renal artery stenosis (Evaluation and management of bilateral renal artery stenosis in children: a case series and review. Pediatr Nephrol 9(3):259-267, 1995).

As a renal fellow at Children's Hospital National Medical Center, in Washington, D.C., in 1987, I developed and published a nephelometric method for the measurement of microalbuminuria. As described in *"Diabetes and the fabulous 'Nephelometer,'"* I used this method to assess the evolution of diabetic kidney disease in a multiyear NIH-sponsored prospective study of individuals with type I diabetes (Pittsburgh Epidemiology of Diabetes Complications study). This study yielded many important observations and resulted in preventive measures that curtail the development of this devastating disorder.

ADMINISTRATION
DEMETRI THE ADMINISTRATOR

IF I PAINTED all experiences in my career as joyful, I am sure I would lose all credibility. And, in fact, some of the circumstances that I am about to divulge provide greater perspective or balance, the yin and the yang, the push and pull, that is the rule rather than the exception in academic medicine.

The moment I accepted the position of director of pediatric nephrology, I became the boss of my secretary, the dialysis nurses and other personnel, nurse specialists, social service worker, dietician, and, of course, all future physicians recruited to assist with the functions of the nephrology division. One of my dreaded chores as the administrator of all these individuals was conducting their annual performance evaluations. In that capacity, I would meet with each individual to discuss their strengths and inadequacies in performing assigned tasks, formulate an action plan to remedy any deficiencies over the subsequent year, and come up with an overall score that translated into practical objectives such as adjustment in salary and job promotion. I then met with an administrator assigned to my division to again discuss all the issues, including the occasional need for termination of employment, and finalize the process.

As a division head, I also had to attend numerous meetings of the department of pediatrics division heads, and with hospital administrators to discuss personnel needs, supplies, and budget to help the nephrology division function efficiently. These meetings enlightened me on the financial aspects of CHP and the University of Pittsburgh, School of Medicine as a whole. Most of these administrative duties were time-consuming and took valuable time away from my more pressing clinical duties, so I became selective about which meetings I would attend. At the same time, I felt guilty for not being better equipped or showing greater enthusiasm for these often-delicate administrative duties, which, for better or worse, were an integral part of my position as the director of pediatric nephrology. Therefore, I tried to be equitable, provide constructive criticism, and also praise the exemplary service of many coworkers.

Realizing that performance reviews are inherently stressful and can damage one's ego as well as one's chances for promotion and salary increase, I made a concerted effort to diffuse stress by using an engaging and sympathetic demeanor, using a soft voice and less adversarial language, and generally try to engender a more pleasant dialogue. This approach seemed to work well, as evidenced by the fact that I did not witness a mass exodus of employees after their performance reviews. But, of course, by their nature, performance reviews are partly subjective and may be perceived differently by management and staff. Performance reviews that resulted in involuntary dismissal or resignation were particularly stressful for me, and probably even more so for the worker. I participated in several such reviews during my career but none as vexing as the dismissal of a senior nephrologist whom I had personally recruited five years earlier. The circumstances described below may prompt the reader to reassess the competence of their own physician.

Starting in early 1993, NG, a then fifty-four-year old professor of pediatric nephrology, began to exhibit signs of forgetfulness and clinical ineptitude. He was a charismatic, gregarious, sociable and handsome man. In short, he was very likable and, at first, other caretakers as well as patients and families were reluctant to submit verbal or written complaints against him. Over the next three years, he exhibited signs of progressive memory loss. He seemed to remember only superficial details about complex patients that the renal team had discussed extensively during patient management conferences. At resident rounds, he offered pathophysiologic scenarios without substantiating his remarks with scientific evidence and listed few details in his patient letter evaluations. I also started to receive complaints at an increasing frequency about the lack of substantive information or disorganized presentations of lectures and informal talks given by NG to pediatric staff and adult nephrology fellows. His teaching and other academic commitments suffered in both amount and content. This led to unfavorable evaluations by medical residents, renal fellows, and students. In addition, despite the provision of protected time to conduct scholarly pursuits, he was unproductive in both his laboratory research and in submitting educational articles for publication in nephrology journals or books.

Toward the end of 1995, NG could not recall giving orders over the telephone to dialysis nurses when contacted at his home during the evenings or overnight. If something questionable or a mishap occurred, the following morning, he would deny having given the order; he simply transferred blame to others. Eventually, this led to consternation and frustration on the part of the dialysis nurses, who expressed to me their lack of confidence in his ability to care for our patients. Soon thereafter, they refused to carry out his orders unless I personally reviewed them, even when I was not on clinical duty. In addition, both written and verbally transmitted complaints about his poor clinical performance were communicated at an increasing rate by multiple individuals, including non-renal nurses, physicians, and families.

As NG's immediate supervisor, I carefully chronicled these complaints as well as deficiencies abstracted directly from patients' clinical records.

I then met with NG, confronted him with the evidence, and asked him to defend several of the more egregious examples of clinical judgment, including grossly inappropriate medication dosages. He immediately became defensive. Rather than a clear and direct reply to my questions, he said, "What would you have done?" I realized that he had used the same phrase repeatedly as a means of concealing or deflecting his inability to provide credible support or a rational explanation for his actions.

At that time, there were only three staff nephrologists in our renal division. Because we shared monthly rotations in the inpatient service equally and we had equal weekend call duty, I had the opportunity to review firsthand the medical records of children managed by this senior nephrologist over the preceding days. In doing so, I noted two striking examples of clinical incompetence. Both occurred during June 1994 and involved younger children managed by peritoneal dialysis who developed peritonitis, a serious infection of the lining of the abdomen and intestines, with virulent bacteria. In both children, the infection led to removal of their peritoneal dialysis catheter, necessitating either replacement of the catheter or temporary conversion to the more cumbersome and invasive form of dialysis-hemodialysis (see pp. 23 and 58). Delay in diagnosis of peritonitis and inappropriate choice and dosage of antibiotic agents likely contributed to this unfortunate chain of events. Of note, one of these bouts of peritonitis occurred four weeks after NG had been chastised for not following the standardized protocol I had devised for managing this complication. His patient notes failed to demonstrate an appreciation of the severity or the urgency of the medical condition, or of the foreseeable consequences and complications stemming from his actions. I identified several other malpractice-like scenarios, which, fortunately, were either averted or of inconsequential harm to the patients. Moreover, I took it upon myself to supervise his clinical work and instructed the ICU and dialysis nurses to notify me with any questionable orders or concerns relating to NG's patient care. All these aspects were reviewed with him and summarized in my annual performance review.

After collecting multiple documents confirming a pattern of poor

REFLECTIONS OF "NEPHRON MAN"

clinical performance and red flags suggesting impaired cognitive function, particularly over the 1993–1994 academic year, I met with the chairman of pediatrics, Dr. Marc Sperling, and the medical director of CHP to seek their counsel and discuss an appropriate course of action. I was advised to continue to document any irregularities and that they would investigate the merits of my concerns. In the meantime, NG spread a rumor among the general pediatric faculty at CHP that I had a personal vendetta against him. He also tried to curb further complaints on my part by accusing me of taking money from families in exchange for accepting their child into our transplant program. In fact, I have always been a goodwill ambassador for our transplant program and encouraged families to come to CHP from abroad and from other parts of the United States. And many did come, not because of bribes that are totally unethical and forbidden by our conflict of interest agreement, but because of our widely publicized excellent graft survival data and high quality of life associated with our unique steroid-sparing tacrolimus monotherapy protocol.

Nonetheless, NG attempted to minimize criticisms of his performance by transferring blame onto me. This became apparent during a meeting in 1995 with the chairman of pediatrics to discuss the issues raised above. The chairman must have been convinced that there was some credibility to his allegations or he simply felt that he had an obligation to formally investigate any allegations, because soon after, I was informed that NG had requested a formal investigation into my own motives. Instead of weighing in the large amount of serious, documented complaints against NG and giving me the benefit of doubt as the division chief, to my surprise and great dismay, the chairman elected to investigate me.

The chairman requested opinions from the heads of several reputable pediatric nephrology programs in the States about my character, professional conduct, and other qualifications. After a few weeks, I was informed by my chairman that that no deficiencies or character faults were noted and that my leadership skills and contributions to our specialty were highly valued. In the interim, NG continued to work at CHP. He was apprised of the results of the investigation of his complaints against me, and given the weight of evidence against him, I suspect that he may have been advised by the chairman to stand down and not make further unfounded accusations. Clearly, NG had become increasingly unhappy with his treatment at CHP and the university. He then resigned from his position, and within one month, he accepted a pediatric staff position at Mercy Hospital of Pittsburgh, a competing local hospital with a small, non-university-affiliated pediatric training program. I am unaware of NG's obligations or duties in connection with that program. Anticipating a negative appraisal from me, NG did not ask me for a reference and probably requested that his new employers not contact me because my report on him would be biased. However, a colleague of NG's at that hospital informed me that, during a lecture on a common nephrologic topic delivered by NG one month after assuming his new job, he became overtly confused and repetitive yet made no apologies and showed no embarrassment. He was then quickly dismissed from that position and soon after was formally diagnosed with a rapidly advancing form of Alzheimer's. Two years later, NG died of complications indirectly attributed to this condition.

NG's circumstances exposed several major flaws in the mind-sets of the hospital administrators and academic medicine leadership at that time. Based on the overwhelming clinical documentation and testimony of multiple caretakers who worked closely with this physician, I naively thought that he would be immediately relieved of all medical duties while investigating the allegations against him. This action would serve our overwhelming priority—preventing harm to the children under our care; from a pragmatic standpoint, this step was also essential in diminishing the malpractice risk for both the physicians and the institution. Yet, to my great astonishment and disappointment, the actions of the CHP leadership suggested that their main priority was assignment of blame. This resulted in exposing children to possible harm while I was being unjustly investigated for bringing attention to NGs suspected mental disorder. If common sense prevailed, NG should have been required to have a formal psycho-behavioral evaluation before he could resume his clinical duties. Instead, it was more expedient to pressure him to resign, rather than endorse indefinite medical leave while maintaining his salary support.

Despite my eventual exoneration in this matter, the investigation of any impropriety on my part was demeaning, stressful, offensive, and inappropriate. It is noteworthy that at that time, I had no recourse because there was no mechanism in place for physicians to request an independent, unbiased assessment of his/her grievances or violation of one's academic rights. Since this incident, CHP and the University of Pittsburgh School of Medicine have made great progress in establishing grievance committees and support groups to ensure fair treatment, strengthen academic freedoms, encourage open disclosure of inappropriate actions or behavior, identify mental impairment that may compromise one's clinical performance, and provide counseling to individuals who believe they have been unfairly targeted by a superior's performance reviews.

MEDICAL MALPRACTICE SUITS: ANATHEMA TO PHYSICIANS

<hr>

HUMAN BEINGS ARE fallible. Thus, decisions made by even the most competent, conscientious, and well-intentioned physicians can occasionally bring harm to their patients. By keeping up with advances in their field and through meticulous and conscientious patient care, one hopes to make as few mistakes as possible over the course of his/her career. Actuarial data indicate that catastrophic complications occur more frequently in fields such as obstetrics and neurosurgery. This accounts for the vastly higher annual malpractice premiums in these specialties. In some instances, the malpractice premiums are so prohibitive as to force physicians to abandon private practice. Apart from factoring in medical liability costs, the threat of being sued has led many physicians to practice a defensive style of medicine. This means ordering numerous, often expensive, and potentially risky tests—even when a common diagnosis suffices, so as not to miss a rare or unexpected condition. As an increasing number of individuals are receiving routine care in emergency departments where their medical history is largely unknown, over-testing is particularly prevalent and is a major contributor to the rapidly rising health care costs in the United States.

Being sued represents an indictment of the doctor's competence and their betrayal of the respect and trust that patients placed in them.

As a group, physicians are caring and empathetic individuals, and when confronted by such suits, more than their ego or reputation is at stake. A long and drawn-out legal process, frivolous charges by a few unscrupulous lawyers and patients, and a popular culture of blaming doctors for years of self-abuse or excesses combine to create a depressing and emotionally stressful experience. Court appearances and a long trial also disrupt a doctor's ability to manage other patients seeking continuity of care. Rather than succumb to the hurdles related to medical malpractice suits, an increasing number of obstetricians in particular have elected to become salaried employees at large medical centers that are well equipped with specialists to manage medical emergencies more effectively and limit the chance for medical errors. In addition, these centers employ teams of qualified lawyers and are in a much better position to negotiate reduced malpractice rates for all physicians under their employment. Unfortunately, this trend has rendered many rural areas underserved in several medical specialties.

Pediatric nephrologists are confronted with seriously ill children nearly on a daily basis. Decisions regarding such complex patients are more likely to result in unintended consequences, prompting possible malpractice suits. Fortunately, during my long career, I have encountered only three suits. None of these required me to testify in court, and no settlement money was paid on my behalf. Nonetheless, as one may surmise from the following anecdote, I found these experiences stressful.

MITIGATING THE RISK FOR MEDICAL MALPRACTICE SUITS

Earlier in this book, I mentioned Mamas in "*Bobby's sad predicament– a paradigm of raw courage and resolve.*" Mamas was a mature and pleasant seventeen-year-old young man who, despite having advanced kidney failure, had a healthy appearance and was an outstanding student. Thus, assuming an uneventful renal transplant, he had every expectation of having good health and a bright and productive future. However, there was no suitable living donor and as his kidney function deteriorated, he developed fluid retention and hypertension, along with biochemical disturbances of a magnitude that met criteria for starting dialysis. Hence, in an elective (nonurgent) procedure, a large-caliber dialysis catheter was placed by an interventional radiologist for initiating hemodialysis. A few hours later, Mamas' began his first dialysis treatment under supervision in the ICU. Within minutes of starting dialysis, his blood pressure fell precipitously, and his breathing became labored. His dialysis nurse informed me that the ICU staff was attending to him. I soon arrived at the ICU and found dozens of ICU personnel, including a cardiac surgeon, actively involved in the resuscitation process. Mamas had received immediate and appropriate treatment but quickly arrested, and despite prolonged efforts, he could not be resuscitated. I recall feeling shaken up and helpless at the gravity of the situation and my inability to contribute any helpful suggestions. I could not even imagine that this was happening. I went into a room about twenty yards away and began to cry inconsolably. I felt that I had somehow betrayed my patient's trust and that this nightmare would not have occurred if I had not recommend starting dialysis. It took me a while to regain my composure. I then faced Mamas' parents in one of the adjoining ICU consulting rooms and explained what we thought had happened and that, sadly, we were not able to save their son.

Later that day, an autopsy revealed that the dialysis catheter had not only penetrated the lumen of the vessel, but also made a tear in the inner lining of the chest wall, or *parietal pleura*. The massive bleeding compressed the outside of the lungs and heart, and together with decreased blood return to the heart, severely compromised heart function and blood pressure support, causing severe oxygen deprivation and death.

My long and close relationship with Mamas and his family made his death extremely painful for me and, of course, it was devastating to his loving parents and siblings. I fully disclosed to Mamas' family that even though this potential perforation and bleeding complication was mentioned by the radiologist and noted on the consent form that they had signed before the procedure, the technical intervention was nevertheless directly responsible for the death of their son. I made a point of detailing in the medical record all the events leading to Mamas' death.

While heartbroken, the family chose not to sue. I will never fully know what went into their decision. Clearly, the family had been pleased with Mamas' quality of medical care over the preceding years and appreciated our strong interpersonal relationship. In addition, they were aware that we had acted in good faith and were forthcoming and honest in admitting our error. In my opinion, these were the most important factors in their decision. Although physicians attend formal seminars that heighten their awareness of medical liability issues and how to avoid or mitigate them, I believe that medical competence and genuine bonding with patients are the best deterrents. Had the circumstances been reversed, I believe that is how physicians would wish to be treated. Far more important to me personally was receiving the family's forgiveness. This was most helpful for my emotional recovery, although this painful memory remains vivid two decades later. Mamas' family however, may never find closure or relief from the pain of losing him, permanently.

MEDICAL RECORD TO THE RESCUE

Ironically, the most memorable medical malpractice suit against me was for perceived inaction, rather than for a harmful intervention. It involved a premature infant whose prenatal ultrasound had revealed severe bilateral multicystic renal disease, a genetic condition in which kidney tissue is largely replaced by nonfunctional, fluid-filled cysts. The presence of only a minimal amount of amniotic fluid volume suggested low urine production and reduced renal function preceding birth. His birth weight was just over four pounds. The infant had lung failure at delivery and required resuscitation followed by mechanical ventilator support. His blood pressure was low, and he had not produced urine. Given the serious renal issues and overall severity of the baby's condition, at about twenty-four hours old, he was transferred from the neonatal unit at Magee Women's Hospital in Pittsburgh to the neonatal ICU at CHP.

I met the family shortly after I reviewed the medical records and examined the baby. Because of the paramount goal to improve the blood pressure and oxygen delivery to all organs, he had received large volumes of saline and had become markedly swollen; his body weight was now nearly eight pounds or double his birth weight. Despite these measures, blood pressure remained low and he required high ventilator settings, suggesting that, in addition to prematurity, he had poorly developed lungs (*pulmonary hypoplasia*), which is commonly associated with low urine production during fetal life. A repeat ultrasound and blood chemistry studies confirmed the presence of the above cystic renal condition and very poor renal function. I then explained to the family that the baby had permanent renal failure. Because of very low and unstable blood pressure, hemodialysis (blood dialysis) was contraindicated. Similarly, peritoneal dialysis (see p.64) was unlikely to aid fluid removal, improve the blood pressure or control blood chemistries. In addition, based on previous experience with a handful of similar challenging cases, I had noted that placement of peritoneal catheters in babies with such degree of skin swelling contributed to infection and hastened their death. Thus, from a medical perspective and on ethical grounds ("do no harm"), I did not recommend starting any form of dialysis. Despite giving a very detailed justification for my decision, the family, perhaps in denial, insisted that everything be done to save their baby. I clearly detailed my recommendations as well as my interactions with the family in the medical record.

A pediatric urologist performed surgery later that evening but was unsuccessful in inserting a catheter to facilitate drainage of the suspected obstructed right ureter. The next day, on the family's insistence, a pediatric renal transplant surgeon was consulted to give an opinion as to the prospect of doing renal transplantation; it was deemed unrealistic in this critically ill premature infant. The baby's condition continued to slowly deteriorate over the next twenty-four hours. By

REFLECTIONS OF "NEPHRON MAN"

Monday morning, my weekend clinical shift had ended, and I gave a medical summary of this patient to a senior staff member who was taking over the clinical service, explaining my reservations about dialysis. Nonetheless, I later learned that the family had persuaded him to intervene. Thus, a peritoneal catheter was placed, but dialysis was ineffective. The baby developed fever and sepsis (infection throughout the body) and died one day later.

Five years later, I received notice of a malpractice suit involving this baby. Despite my limited contact with his family over that weekend, the indictment was twelve pages long and enumerated fifty-four counts in which the lawyers for the plaintiff had found me negligent. The hospital lawyers informed me that this was a common tactic; the overwhelming number of complaints were intended to induce shock and a sense of culpability, rather than represent the facts. The hospital, the urologist, and other physicians involved in the baby's care were also sued. In my view, the suit was unjustifiable (perhaps even ridiculous), but the implications for CHP and I were serious.

Late one morning, I was summoned to give a deposition along with several other colleagues. The room was small and cramped with four imposing lawyers for the plaintiff and two from CHP, a legal clerk taking a shorthand account, a professional videographer, a CHP administrator, and myself. I was asked to go over the indictment point-by-point and explain my notes from five years earlier. To refresh my memory, they presented me with their copy of the copious medical records that were generated during the relatively brief time the baby was under our care. Parenthetically, a rule of thumb of mine is: If the medical records in paper form outweigh the child, the prognosis is dismal. In fact, I recalled the case well and had had the chance to review my original notes prior to the deposition. The most contentious point was: Dr. Ellis, why did you delay and did not perform dialysis which could have saved the baby? I replied that I had clearly explained to the family that, in my expert opinion, the high risks associated with this procedure far outweighed any possible benefits. To my surprise, the plaintiff's lead lawyer disputed my answer and insisted that there was no such documentation in their copy of the medical record. I was surprised and incredulous that my note from the first night after admission to CHP was missing. I then requested to see the original patient records, which were in front of me on the table, and lo and behold, my note was there. I read it slowly and loudly for everyone to hear, and for the camera. Then, I went on the offensive and asked how such a key note was missing in their copy of the medical records. "Was this intentional?" I asked with a slightly annoyed voice. There was no reply. "If the baby died after I performed dialysis, I would have committed an unethical act bordering on malpractice," I continued. At this point, the plaintiff lawyers glanced at each other and appeared visibly embarrassed. They did not have any further questions for me. I was then quickly dismissed and never heard from them again. I believe that my testimony was instrumental in the family's decision to drop the entire suit against CHP.

This case illustrates the importance of writing detailed and meticulous patient progress notes and to be totally transparent in disclosing any errors that have harmed or could have harmed a child. Discovery of hidden or concealed medical errors is rarely, if ever, forgiven by patients and is likely to augment punitive damages. I have utilized this story repeatedly to reinforce these lessons with our younger faculty, residents and fellows.

Medicine and Politics

―――❦―――

"A MEETING IS an organized way of prolonging decisions or justifying one's job," Demetrius Ellis.

From the onset, I must confess that, for as long as I can remember, I have always had a strong antipathy for any politics. This is contrary to my Greek heritage and the unfounded notion that every Greek has the gene for philosophy and politics. Perhaps, I am the exception to this rule. Therefore, one may summarily disqualify me from commenting on politics with one possible exception: medical politics with which I have a modest amount of first-hand experience. In relation to health care, it is well-known that a major function of government is to legislate measures that make medical care more affordable and accessible to all citizens, ensure the quality of care, reduce abuses of Medicare and overbilling by hospitals and private providers, protect the drug and food supply of the nation, and curtail the rapidly rising cost of medical care. However, while I support these missions, I have had personal encounters with government agencies that utilized unnecessarily aggressive and counterproductive tactics to achieve these objectives. I contend that the events recounted herein support the charge that, while well-intended, the actions of government officials directly resulted in more than doubling in the cost of renal transplants in children at CHP without a substantive improvement in transplant outcome.

As medical director of pediatric renal transplantation at CHP for over thirty-five years, I helped pioneer immunosuppression regimens that have served children well for nearly forty years (see "Personal research contributions"). Under my supervision and as required by Medicare, transplant results from our center were submitted on a timely basis to several transplant registries. These include the government-sponsored Scientific Registry of Transplant Recipients (SRTR) and its contractual agency, United Network Organ Sharing (UNOS). We also cooperated with the local Center for Organ Recovery and Education (CORE). In addition, we voluntarily participated in the acclaimed nongovernmental North American Pediatric Renal Transplant Cooperative Study (NAPRTCS). Moreover, CHP's patient and kidney transplant or graft survival data as well as special quality of life measures were described in several journal articles authored by me and by other members of our renal transplant program. The results were exemplary, and therefore, CHP's management protocol had been replicated in other pediatric transplant programs worldwide. In fact, the outcomes were particularly striking given that CHP's transplant program was more willing to accept high-risk candidates, some of whom were rejected by other prestigious institutions. However, during the period from May 20, 2006, to June 24, 2009, our kidney transplant success rate (allograft survival rate [ASR]) fell to 85%, which was just below the lower nationally accepted limit of 87%. Given the fact that, like other pediatric transplant programs, we performed a relatively small number of renal transplants (fifteen to twenty annually), this would not have triggered any alarms if we had one less transplant failure during the time in question. Of course, we agonized over each individual child that lost their kidney and scrutinized these vexing failures during our weekly renal rounds and in our mandatory monthly transplant quality council meetings.

On review of the causes of graft loss, we noted that one resulted from accidental vascular injury related to a biopsy done at interventional radiology. A second graft loss occurred in an infant who died at home because of a previously unidentified cardiac disorder; the graft actually functioned well, but it is technically counted as a loss. The other losses were deemed unavoidable and occurred in patients with high levels of circulating antibodies and clinical features predictive of high risk for graft failure, such as previous kidney transplant loss because of rejection. We fully disclosed all incidental and accidental graft losses to the families and the reporting agencies. In any case, despite a graft survival rate of 100% in 2005 and superior historical allograft survival rates in 2006 as well as during the two years between June 2009, and June 2011, the substandard 85% results noted in June, 2009 put us under radar-scrutiny by the Centers for Medicare and Medicaid Services (CMS). Among many other functions, this governmental agency oversees the quality of care and confers payment to transplant programs. In my opinion, the intended and unintended consequences stemming from the actions of CMS representatives were far-reaching and, to some measure, irresponsible or unjustified.

Instead of taking a pragmatic, common-sense approach to these legitimate, substandard kidney transplant outcome results at our center, CMS issued a detailed Systems Improvement Agreement (SIA), a legal document intended to aid compliance with the Conditions of Participation in federal programs. This SIA stated that CMS would continue to operate and fund our program for one year under probation with scrutiny and supervision by the CMS staff, to ascertain that all remedial actions were fully implemented. The implicit threat was that if the renal transplant program did not adhere to every aspect of the SIA agreement, they would stop payments to our program (see p. 19, Law 92-603). Furthermore, by association, this probationary period extended to all programs at CHP, including heart, liver, lung, and gastrointestinal transplants, even though there were no performance concerns related to these programs. Because Medicare funded over 90% of our transplants, a decision by CMS to rescind such payments posed a threat to the very existence of CHP's transplant program. Apart from imposing a devastating financial blow and damaging the reputation of

CHP and the University of Pittsburgh, such CMS action could potentially shut down our entire transplant program. More importantly, anything that undermined the transplant program, could jeopardize the very lives of all children in Western Pennsylvania in urgent need of this procedure.

By their admission, CMS administrators assigned to enforce the SIA recommendations were unfamiliar with the common urologic and medical conditions that could influence the outcome of pediatric renal transplantation and showed little interest in validating the mitigating factors described in our detailed case-by-case review or consider the "multiple proportional hazards models" that could explain our temporary suboptimal ASR results.

To guide the interaction between our transplant administrators and those from CMS, CHP immediately retained a high-priced lawyer uniquely experienced with several adult hospitals that had overcome similar SIAs. Numerous meetings ensued and consumed a lot of time on the part of many administrators and medical personnel who attended. There were prolonged discussions about the choice of words and phrases of the initial SIA and the many qualifying conditions imposed over the ensuing year. The tone, language, and demeanor employed by the CMS staff were not ones of reconciliation and cooperation; instead, they made it abundantly clear that they were in charge and the undisputed champions of these highly unproductive and extremely costly skirmishes. Their actions were an affront and caused stress and anxiety to me and to the outstanding surgeons, nurses, and administrators at CHP who worked diligently to achieve the exemplary kidney transplant outcomes obtained over the nearly three preceding decades.

Over those three decades, CHP had committed substantial financial resources, time, and effort to developing its overall transplant program, which eventually became its crown jewel. Hence, the transplant administrators who spearheaded the negotiations on the part of CHP made many concessions to CMS, rather than risk losing all they had built over many years; it was imperative to demonstrate complete compliance with each aspect of the SIA, regardless of validity of the demands or financial burden to CHP.

One mandate of the SIA was that each family whose child was on the renal transplant waiting list would receive a letter informing them of our suboptimal results compared to data from other pediatric centers. Each family was then given the option to undergo a transplant evaluation and re-listing of their child at another institution of their choice with all pertinent expenses paid by CHP. One requirement that did make a lot of sense was to have a team of pediatric nephrology and surgery experts from reputable institutions perform a thorough independent peer review of each failure, as well as conduct interviews with all professional staff and an inspection of our facilities. Their written independent assessments would then be sent to both CMS and to CHP. Because improving transplant survival was the primary objective of both CMS and CHP, we welcomed a comprehensive review. As it turned out, the eventual peer review findings exonerated our program and praised our in-house remediation efforts stemming from our extensive internal patient management reviews. In fact, we had already addressed and remedied various deficiencies well before CMS became involved in reviewing our program. Yet, despite this favorable review and its mandate to reduce Medicare costs, CMS required us to hire multiple additional personnel to implement their directives. As a result, CHP had to assume the cost of hiring a quality process improvement specialist, three dedicated renal transplant nurse coordinators, a data input person, a quality program administrator, full-time rather than part-time social worker, dietician and behavioral psychologist and other personnel, each requiring office space, furniture, computers, etc. This substantially and permanently raised the cost for transplantation, making our center less financially competitive compared to other pediatric renal transplant programs. Apparently, CMS did not weigh-in the fact that, compared to adult transplant programs, pediatric hospitals perform relatively few transplants and, therefore, are much less able to absorb the high cost associated with redundant regulations that often penalize highly successful programs.

The irony is that many of the above legitimate concerns could have been resolved in a more efficient, much less costly, and more amicable manner. As a first step, CMS could have assigned the independent peer review team described above to review the merits of any potential performance infractions, before issuing a SIA. CMS must recognize that mitigating circumstances and occasional "perfect storms" can occur at any center. A more respectful, collegial, and cooperative, rather than threatening, interaction would have been far more appropriate. Second, CMS should have been much more cognizant of the costs to an institution resulting from their mandates. This is especially important when permanent job positions are requested by CMS that hospitals cannot afford. Third, the transplant and quality initiatives administrator of CMS charged with reviewing a program should have greater familiarity with the basic aspects of transplantation; this would make his/her arguments more realistic and credible to hospital personnel. Fourth, every effort should be made to eliminate or consolidate under one umbrella all overlapping tasks currently performed at great cost by multiple overseeing agencies. Regulatory policies are also extremely cumbersome and need to be streamlined to improve compliance and care. Such efficiency improvements may have a significant economic benefit and also optimize transplant outcomes.

My crisis in academic medicine: a story of, "David vs. Goliath"

<hr/>

DURING THE COURSE of a long career, nearly everyone will encounter challenging situations that compel them to defend their convictions and take altruistic actions even at the risk of putting their livelihood in peril. Because of their firm belief in the ethical principle of "do no harm" first advanced by Hippocrates, also known as "nonmaleficence", or "primum non nocere" in Latin meaning, "first do no harm", physicians take a strong stance on issues pertaining to patient welfare and safety. Such unwavering responses on the part of doctors go a long way in solidifying the trust and respect between patients and their physicians. Thus, it is the duty of physicians and other caretakers to promptly report medical errors or medical practices that they perceive to be harmful to patients. Many states have enacted laws mandating such reporting and agencies such as the Joint Commission use this as a criterion for hospital accreditation. Thus, health care facilities have special committees that convene at a moment's notice to review accidents and medical errors. By promoting transparency and awareness and finding means for reducing or effectively managing errors, these practices focus on patient safety rather than casting blame on the perpetrator. In fact, physicians acting in good faith are protected by the Whistleblower Protection Act against reprisals from employers who may stand to lose funds and reputation because of public disclosure of egregious violations or practices. Under such a protective umbrella, the risk to physicians reporting patient safety concerns nowadays is negligible and rarely reaches crisis proportions or affect one's professional future. However, this was not the case in the personal story I am about to relate.

My crisis took place early in my career, before the existence of several of the above formal reporting and regulatory mechanisms. It emerged from my concerns over perceived suboptimal care of children undergoing transplantation at my hospital. What began as a simple, well-intentioned and worthwhile endeavor, evolved into a crisis with potentially profound consequences for me, my family and my patients. It pitted me, "David," against Dr. Thomas Starzl and several of his hospital and university backers, "Goliath". In fact, my decision to place patient interests above my own, tested my resolve, strength of character and integrity; it also had detrimental effects on my mental and physical health. However, upon reflecting back on my career, unequivocally, taking such a decisive action, represents my most important patient contribution. In retrospect, this was the most inspiring and proud event in my life, as well as a source of lasting professional satisfaction and fulfillment. Thus, although I could choose to put behind and not share with you any of these unfortunate and painful bygone events, several reasons compel me to so. First and foremost, the story gives a greater perspective of the limited autonomy physicians employed at major academic centers exert over their professional decisions as compared to doctors who are in control of their own medical practice. Importantly, this account also raises awareness among young physicians of unanticipated encounters that may also compel them that to make career-defining choices, should they pursue a similar academic path.

In the microcosm of academic medicine, the explosive growth of the transplantation program at the University of Pittsburgh and UPMC starting in 1981 was, in my view, truly transformative. The single most important individual spearheading this program was Dr. Thomas Starzl. Prior to 1981, apart of kidney transplants, organ transplantation was markedly curtailed because of ineffective or toxic immunosuppressive agents and, to a lesser degree, by surgical impediments. Dr. Starzl had just received exclusive approval to conduct clinical trials of a new, more promising immunosuppressive agent - cyclosporine. Preliminary studies indicated that this agent had the potential to revolutionize transplantation of all organs. This, together with Dr. Starzl's innovative surgical technique with liver transplantation, made him an outstanding prospect for recruitment at any prestigious center. His longtime friend, Dr. Henry T. Bahnson, chief of surgery at UPMC, and the then acting dean of the University of Pittsburgh, School of Medicine, Dr. Thomas Detre, were great visionaries and realized the potential value of recruiting Dr. Starzl from Denver, Colorado. If cyclosporine proved to be as effective as they hoped, the sky would be the limit for Dr. Starzl and for the University of Pittsburgh, School of Medicine.

Seemingly instantaneously, Dr. Starzl and cyclosporine gave Pittsburgh a huge competitive edge in transplantation, almost a monopoly. Because of the huge global backlog of patients in dire need of a variety of organ transplants, liver in particular, this program grew exponentially. Within three to four years, nearly all the expectations and predictions surrounding cyclosporine and the transplant program under Dr. Starzl's leadership were not only realized but exceeded. Thus, "Dr. Starzl's transplant program", generated much income and prestige and quickly became the crown jewel of the University of Pittsburgh, School of Medicine. In addition to generous support from Sandoz Pharmaceutical Co. the developer of cyclosporine, moneys poured in at an unprecedented rate from multiple government-sponsored research sources, hospital development foundations, and private donors who were eager to support all activities associated with this highly visible program that all the media branded as, "the miracle of life." In addition to a massive building boom, these funds, enabled the recruitment of many renowned clinicians and researchers in multiple fields sub-serving transplantation. These highly visible and prestigious achievements catapulted the University of Pittsburgh, School of Medicine and UPMC high in the national university rankings; indeed, Dr. Starzl was the undisputed single most important asset of our university. Notably, he was fully aware of his value and how to leverage it. In addition, his self-esteem and ego were boosted by the many praises he received from his grateful patients. Making possible the "gift of life" was nothing short of miraculous. In fact, the transplant program grew so big as to have a tangible effect on the economy of the entire city of Pittsburgh, where "Tom Starzl" became a household name. Hence, it is not surprising that he was accorded preferential treatment that included generous financial resources and liberal authority in leading the transplant program. Such accessions to single physicians of superstar-status seemed to be more prevalent at many hospitals and universities at that time. Under these prevailing conditions, it became very difficult for hospital administrators or university leaders to resist Dr. Starzl's demands because displeasing him could result in his relocation at another institution. In summary, multiple factors converged to create a perfect storm and enable Dr. Starzl to become extremely powerful and influential.

It is noteworthy that although the transplant program had many great attributes, one important detraction was that the working relationship between Dr. Starzl and other key participants was not as harmonious as one may be led to believe. There were several physicians, such as myself, who were swept up by the transplantation tsunami at UPMC.

I became well acquainted with Dr. Starzl through my interactions with mutual patients and had many private and group meetings with him over the years. He was intelligent, charismatic, and passionate about his work. He was also authoritative, tended to micromanage, and demanded unquestionable loyalty from everyone remotely connected to the transplant program. Trainees and staff physicians who did not question his opinions and guidance were rewarded with strong recommendations for employment at prestigious institutions seeking to initiate their own transplant programs. In contrast, those who questioned his decisions could face his wrath or even dismissal. Consequently, many physicians and administrative personnel acquiesced to Dr. Starzl's demands, rather than risk their careers and reputations. While I empathized with those making such pragmatic choices I realized that repeated capitulation to Dr. Starzl's demands only led to an even more authoritarian approach to patient management. Thus, he often dismissed input by medical consultants and colleagues that may well have contributed to better clinical management decisions. Intentionally or otherwise, on occasion, his actions directly harmed the mental and physical health of several co-workers, including me.

I allege that important safety concerns surrounding the use of cyclosporine were not adequately addressed or were ignored by the leadership overseeing the transplant program. It was as though success with preventing rejection and effectuating survival of the transplanted organ, rather than the patient, was the ultimate objective. As such, Dr. Starzl insisted on maintaining high blood cyclosporine levels. This issue put me in direct conflict with him. Because the chronology and the sensitivity of background information are important in judging the validity of my allegations or conclusions, I ask the reader's indulgence as I review the timing and substance of key incidents. More detailed information supporting my story are beyond the scope of this book but can be found in several newspaper articles that were published during the period in question.

At the time Dr. Starzl was appointed chief of solid organ transplantation at the University of Pittsburgh and UPMC, there existed a robust and relatively successful renal transplant program under the senior leadership of Dr. Thomas Hakala, a renowned adult urologist. This service had conducted all the previous pediatric renal transplants at CHP, and I and my pediatric nephrology staff played a major role in all preoperative and postoperative care of these children. This was an amicable and effective partnership in part because nearly half of our mutual pediatric patients had urological disorders as the cause of their renal failure and benefited by the concurrent urological/nephrology expertise. However, upon his arrival, Dr. Starzl set up a separate general transplant surgery service under his direct leadership. This service performed only a few pediatric kidney transplants and involved multiple rather than one or two assigned surgeons. This limited the ability of any single surgeon to accrue sufficient expertise in pediatric renal transplantation. Such expertise gap widened as the number of transplant surgeons quickly exceeded fifty. Yet, training in pediatric renal transplantation was essential for accreditation of graduates of the newly established Thomas E. Starzl Transplantation Institute Fellowship Program. Many of these surgeons were very capable but had little or no pediatric or urologic experience. Thus, they had very limited expertise with perioperative fluid and electrolyte management, poor knowledge of pharmacologic choices and dosages, and little familiarity with psycho-behavioral issues unique to the pediatric population. These concerns impelled me to become more proactive in averting medical complications especially when several zealous but very inexperienced surgical residents and fellows sought to take charge of my patients.

This brings me to the most contentious issue, the use of cyclosporine itself. Apart from a preliminary study that had been published by Sir Roy Y. Calne in England in 1981 showing very promising results in adult renal transplant recipients, Dr. Starzl was the only investigator to receive approval by the Food and Drug Administration to conduct initial trials of cyclosporine in the United States. Because cyclosporine was a new and very powerful agent, and clinical experience in humans was very limited at that time, a learning curve to determine its efficacy and adverse effects was inevitable. Based on the available research, Dr. Starzl had arrived at a starting oral dose capable of meeting the essential requirement, namely, adequate immunosuppression capable of preventing organ rejection. The patient was then closely monitored for clinical and biochemical toxicity related to the drug, as well as assessment of the degree of immunosuppression and occurrences of rejection.

However, it became quickly clear that there existed a significant variation in the metabolism of cyclosporine among patients. Thus, a fixed or standard drug dosage did not result in predictable or uniform drug blood levels and, therefore, did not correlate with the desired degree of immunosuppression. Therefore, rejection rates could vary markedly from one individual to the next. We then deduced and confirmed that by adjusting the drug dosage such as to raise the blood level above certain limits, we achieved greater acceptance of the organ. However, these blood levels were not based on any systematic study. Moreover, the therapeutic and toxic blood concentration range appeared especially narrow in children compared to adults, even after adjusting for variations in age and body size. Thus, predictably, children with blood cyclosporine levels at the higher end of this arbitrary target range began to exhibit multiple systemic short- and long-term side effects some of which were potentially life-threatening. Despite the clear indications of drug toxicity, Dr. Starzl fiercely enforced these high goal levels. In fact, he remained steadfast and uncompromising over the next five years despite accruing experience at other centers demonstrating better transplant outcomes than ours, while utilizing blood target levels of cyclosporine that were 60-80 percent lower than ours. These centers also reported fewer serious neurologic symptoms, such as extremity or finger tremors, insomnia, depression, and severe headaches, all of which were quite common in our patients. Younger children at our center also had a much higher incidence of posttransplant lymphoproliferative disease (PTLD), a serious but largely reversible premalignant lymphoma-like disorder triggered by Epstein-Barr virus (EBV), as well as other hematologic and infectious complications attributed to excessive immunosuppression. Moreover, our patients routinely encountered facial hair growth and perceptible enlargement of the gums, and many had transient diabetes mellitus, high blood pressure requiring one or more agents to control, and kidney toxicity manifest by reduced renal function. This was important because in renal transplant recipients it raised concern about rejection that may have led to further increases, rather than decreases, in cyclosporine dosages, thereby resulting in greater toxicity. Furthermore, medical noncompliance was decidedly more prevalent among adolescent females who developed facial hair and other disfiguring side effects related to cyclosporine. In fact, four of these girls admitted to such non-compliance which led to rejection and eventual kidney loss. Rather than embrace and rectify this psychologically-based underlying cause of rejection in this pediatric sub-population, Dr. Starzl's focus seemed to be exclusively set on the kidney transplant survival rate.

Based on our own experience and mounting new data from several other institutions, I was totally convinced that many of the complications could be curtailed or avoided altogether through judicious reduction of cyclosporine blood levels. Not only did Dr. Starzl disagree, but he offered no plausible explanation. I can only surmise that he was convinced that he was uniquely capable of determining these levels for individual organ recipients, even though there was no systematic effort to reach a specific therapeutic drug range, other than universally high blood levels. Thus, to the chagrin and dismay of other senior physicians, Dr. Starzl personally interdicted and reversed their orders to lower cyclosporine dosages in patients experiencing toxic effects. I made concerted efforts and pleaded with him in hopes of persuading him to change his mind. These same contentious patient safety concerns related to cyclosporine use were widely prevalent throughout all other transplant services at CHP. However, reporting my concerns to outside agencies as "medical errors or mistaken drug use" was not an option for me, particularly if the side effects represented non-fatal events or near misses, also known as "sentinel", errors. These could not be proven given the absence of well conducted and published scientific studies describing a consensus approach to cyclosporine use and what constitutes unacceptable health risks-side effects- specifically in the pediatric renal transplantation population. However, confronted with these ongoing issues and the apparent impasse with Dr. Starzl, I came to the inescapable conclusion that I had a moral obligation to my pediatric patients and their families who entrusted them to me, to take a more decisive stand.

As a first step, in May 1986, I performed a detailed review and analysis of our overall renal transplant experience. I reasoned that this would enable me to more precisely document the frequency and severity of the perceived side effects associated with the cyclosporine regimen as well as examine the surgical complications, and thereby offer fact-based, pragmatic suggestions aimed at improving patient outcomes. By 1986, we had by far the largest series to date, consisting of seventy-two children. Most of the transplants were performed by the adult urology transplant surgery. Dr. Starzl was involved mostly with liver and multi-visceral transplantation and was the surgeon on record in only five cases while eleven additional kidney transplants were performed by his subordinates on the general transplant surgery team. Our aggregate kidney survival rate after one year was modest, at about 60% compared with more than 80% elsewhere. Moreover, our data fully supported my contention that most of the important complications and the substandard renal allograft survival results were primarily related to excessive immunosuppression.

Armed with these compelling data, I arranged to meet with Dr. Starzl in the hopes of discussing strategies for improving our results. For purposes of comparison, I compiled several just published journal articles comprising small pediatric renal transplant series from other centers. After a cursory glance at the front page of each article, Dr. Starzl selectively read out the names of the authors several of whom were his former trainees. Apart from this, he paid little attention to the content of the articles and quickly tossed them back on the pile. This dismissive attitude, suggested that his former students and trainees possessed no knowledge than that he had imparted to them. He contended that their "better results" were not related to their modified immunosuppression protocol and concluded that their series of patients must have included healthier children with fewer co-morbidities or less complex conditions.

Although I was in total disbelief at Dr. Starzl's quick dismissal of all the evidence I had painstakingly collected, I elected to put my personal annoyance aside and chose a non-confrontational and diplomatic approach in hopes of persuading him that our results together with my review of the literature strongly supported the following conclusions:

Our higher rate of complications and suboptimal renal allograft failure rates were largely related to,

1. Excessive use of immunosuppression, i.e., cyclosporine,
2. Inappropriate choice of donated kidneys, such as the combined use of both small kidneys mostly transplanted by members of the urology transplant staff, that led to prolonged hospital stay, and higher surgical complication rates eventually resulting in organ failure and high death rate.
3. Dr. Starzl's unique and unsubstantiated stand of not accepting living donor kidneys from willing parents, leading some families to pursue their child's transplant elsewhere. (Several published pediatric series later confirmed a clear advantage of living donor kidneys especially in infants and younger children. (See Kidney Int in 1986 by Su, Mauer, Simmons and Nigarian et al. from Minnesota; and data from the very large transplant registry, North American Pediatric Renal Transplant-Trials Cooperative-Collaborative Study-Studies, NAPRTCS established in 1987).
4. Performance of transplants by physicians who were inexperienced and also had minimal general pediatric surgical training, thus compromising many aspects of care during and immediately after the transplant. (This implied that designating one to two competent surgeons to perform pediatric kidney transplants could improve our transplant outcomes.)

The solution to each of these substantive components was easily deduced and very feasible. Dr. Starzl promised to consider my suggestions. This raised my hopes that substantive changes would be forthcoming, particularly in our cyclosporine regimen.

Three months after this meeting, the stalemate over immunosuppression and other concerns persisted. Moreover, my attempts to obtain additional transplant data from the transplant office that would enabled me to confirm and reconcile a few discrepancies and complete my ongoing data analysis, were ignored. Thus, on October 6, 1986, I decided to take a calculated gamble and send a confidential memorandum directly to Dr. Starzl for the express purpose of spurring action. In it, I reminded him of the issues discussed at our previous meeting in May 1986 and expressed my frustration over the lack of any progress. I stated that I was declaring a moratorium on pediatric renal transplantation at CHP until I had received assurances that my concerns were adequately addressed and that specific changes will be implemented. The sealed envelope containing the memorandum was hand delivered to Dr. Starzl's office by my trusted secretary.

On Monday morning, October 13, 1986, I received a telephone call from two investigative reporters of *The Pittsburgh Press*, Mrs. Flaherty and Mr. Schneider. I was shocked to learn that they had specific information contained in my memorandum. Of course, I did not deny writing it and attested to the validity of the contents. The reporters would not disclose their informant but had several questions regarding my allegations. Because I knew that I had not misstated the deficiencies of the transplant program in my memo and because the inadvertent disclosure of my concerns had the potential to force corrective action from the transplant service, I provided brief, unexaggerated answers to their questions.

The following morning, Tuesday, October 14, 1986, just before 7:00 a.m., our home telephone rang. Upon answering, I heard the deep voice of the newly appointed medical director of CHP, Dr. Donaldson. He said, "What did you do?" "I hope that you have tenure," he continued. "You put us in a lot of trouble. You can't do that! Have you seen this morning's *Pittsburgh Press*?" I confessed I had not, and he then informed me that a front-page article had reprinted excerpts of my October 6 confidential memo to Dr. Starzl. I was expected in Dr.

Donaldson's office at 8:00 a.m., as an urgent meeting had been convened to discuss the "crisis." I took a quick shower, dressed, and despite the morning traffic, I arrived at the meeting on time. This was the beginning of what turned out to be a prolonged and very stressful ordeal for me and, by extension, for my family.

Already present in Dr. Donaldson's office were the acting chairman of pediatrics, Dr. James R. Zuberbuhler, chief of cardiology; Dr. Mark Rowe, surgeon-in-chief at CHP; and, of course, Dr. Starzl. Also present were two highly respected senior pediatricians; Dr. Richard Michaels, chief of infectious diseases and Dr. Paul Gaffney, chief of the pediatric diagnostic group. I was well acquainted with these latter individuals and respected them immensely. Their presence and warm greeting gave me comfort as I encountered the displeased faces of the others in the room who seemed to avoid eye contact with me.

On the mahogany conference table was the article from *The Pittsburgh Press*, written by Mrs. Flaherty and Mr. Schneider. The prominent headline on the first page read "Presby pediatric kidney transplants draw fire." This extensive and well-written article, accurately reflected my transplant concerns. They had also interviewed other faculty involved with the pediatric renal transplant program, many of whom shared my concerns. Specifically, the article stated, "Ellis questioned the expertise level of the surgeons doing the children's transplants, the drug programs used in treatment, and the quality of donor kidneys, particularly whether they were stored too long or were physically damaged." In addition, it stated, "The chief kidney specialist at Children's Hospital says he will not allow surgeons at Presbyterian-University Hospital to perform any more kidney transplants on his patients until the surgeons assure him that the quality of care will be improved."

Pittsburgh Press, October 14, 1986

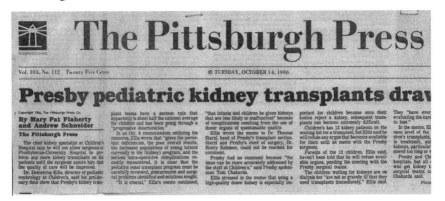

The Pittsburgh Press

Vol. 103, No. 112   Twenty Five Cents   © TUESDAY, OCTOBER 14, 1986

Presby pediatric kidney transplants drav

Copyright 1986, The Pittsburgh Press Co.

**By Mary Pat Flaherty
and Andrew Schneider**

The Pittsburgh Press

The chief kidney specialist at Children's Hospital says he will not allow surgeons at Presbyterian-University Hospital to perform any more kidney transplants on his patients until the surgeons assure him that the quality of care will be improved.

Dr. Demetrius Ellis, director of pediatric nephrology at Children's, said his preliminary data show that Presby's kidney trans-plant teams have a success rate that apparently is about half the national average for children and has been going through a "progressive deterioration."

In an Oct. 6 memorandum outlining his concerns, Ellis wrote that "given the persistent deficiencies, the poor overall results, the increased populations of young infants currently in the (kidney) program, and the serious intra-operative complications recently encountered, it is clear that the pediatric renal transplant program must be carefully reviewed, procurement and surgical problems identified and solutions sought.

"It is crucial," Ellis's memo continued, "that infants and children be given kidneys that are less likely to malfunction" because of complications resulting from the use of donor organs of questionable quality.

Ellis wrote the memo to Dr. Thomas Starzl, head of Presby's transplant section. Starzl and Presby's chief of surgery, Dr. Henry Bahnson, could not be reached for comment.

Presby had no comment because "the issue can be more accurately addressed by the staff at Children's," said Presby spokesman Tom Chakurda.

Ellis stressed in the memo that using a high-quality donor kidney is especially im-portant for children because once their bodies reject a kidney, subsequent transplants can become extremely difficult.

Children's has 12 kidney patients on the waiting list for a transplant, but Ellis said he will refuse any organ that becomes available for them until he meets with the Presby surgeons.

Parents of the 12 children, Ellis said, haven't been told that he will refuse available organs, pending the meeting with the Presby surgical teams.

The children waiting for kidneys are on dialysis but "are not so gravely ill that they need transplants immediately," Ellis said.

They "have ever evaluating the care to lose."

In the memo, El ence level of the dren's transplants, in treatment, and kidneys, particular stored too long or w

Presby and Chi hospitals, but all who get kidney t surgical teams co Chakurda said.

Pleas

After I sat down, Dr. Donaldson asked, "Do you know who leaked the memorandum to the press?" I had no idea and told him as much. "What possessed you to write the memo, and on whose authority did you unilaterally declare a moratorium on pediatric renal transplantation?"

I explained the events leading to my decision and expressed my frustration over the lack of progress surrounding my concerns. I confessed to feeling a moral and ethical obligation to improve the clinical outcome of my patients. A memo seemed to be a reasonable way to clearly articulate my concerns and suggestions, point by point, in the hope of eliciting changes; my loyalty to CHP was unquestionable. I expressed regrets that my concerns and initiatives were exposed publicly. I suggested interrogating Dr. Starzl's office staff for the leak and then briefly reviewed the chronology and content of my previous correspondence with Dr. Starzl, along with my review of our own transplant data, which I had brought with me. Although it was evident that I had made a concerted effort to substantiate my complaints, forbidding a surgeon of Dr. Starzl's stature to perform renal transplants on my patients was viewed as disrespectful and certain to provoke a press frenzy.

Apparently, Reuters, Associated Press, and many television news stations in and outside of Pittsburgh were already calling the CHP press office for updates. Thus, attention shifted towards countermeasures to protect our public relations image rather than focus on my allegations concerning transplant and health safety issues. Dr. Donaldson asked for suggestions on "how should we go about this while we address Ellis's concerns institutionally?"

Dr. Starzl offered the following statement for release to the press: "Dr. Ellis met with Drs. Starzl, Donaldson, and other leadership staff of CHP. It was concluded that Dr. Ellis was unauthorized and premature in declaring a moratorium on pediatric renal transplantation. However, all the issues that he raised in his memorandum will be reviewed and addressed in a timely fashion." Several reasons went into my decision to agree to this press release. First, I had received assurances from all those attending the meeting that our transplant data would be independently authenticated by Dr. Richard Michaels, as to resolve the contentious issues and proceed with transplanting children without further delay. In addition, my overriding objective was to resolve the above transplant problems and not to create controversy or tarnish the reputation of CHP. We were to reconvene at an unspecified future date to discuss Dr. Michaels's findings and come up with mutually acceptable recommendations.

Subsequent articles in *The Pittsburgh Press* and *Post-Gazette* on October 15, 1986 reflected the public relations stance that we had mutually agreed upon during our meeting on the previous morning. Additional quotes for the press and television media were furnished mainly by Dr. Starzl and, in addition to portraying a harmonious transplant team with a unified purpose, these press releases also downplayed our lower success outcomes by citing several plausible but impertinent explanations.

Similarly, on October 16, 1986, a live press conference was held at the spacious hospital cafeteria at CHP. This was attended by a large gathering of CHP physicians, representative of CHP leadership staff, and others who wished to learn the facts surrounding this controversy directly from those involved. Some came anticipating a high-noon-like duel between me and Dr. Starzl, or David and Goliath. Instead of the expected spectacle, they heard me say: "We met and discussed the issues raised in my memorandum, and I am confident and satisfied that genuine efforts were already in progress to review our transplant results and to remedy any deficiencies." Even though I stood by the poor recent outcome results confirmed by my own analysis, I said there was no de facto moratorium and that I could not offer any comments on the validity of several points in my memorandum until all data were analyzed, and that, in fact, an analysis was forthcoming. Furthermore, I added, "My use of the word *moratorium* was possibly inappropriate. What I meant was that renal transplantation will not take place until the data was analyzed." Dr. Starzl spoke after me in a soft, conciliatory tone. He stated, "Dr. Ellis had no ill intentions and has no reservations about referring his patients for transplantation."

In April 1987, Dr. Michaels presented a written report of his independent review, which were identical to mine. In the interim, a prominent pediatric nephrologist from the University of Minnesota, Dr. Michael Mauer, had been invited to examine the validity of my concerns, provide an independent assessment of the renal transplant program at CHP, and contribute his recommendations. His formal review was never shared with me and there was no mention of any action based on the reviews and recommendations of both Drs. Michaels and Mauer. A year after the publication of my memo in *The Pittsburgh Press*, business proceeded as usual—absolutely nothing had been done to remedy the care of our transplant patients.

The period between October 14, 1986, and April 1987 was very stressful for me, both physically and emotionally. I had devoted years to achieving the highest competency level within my discipline and bettering the care of my patients, even sacrificing time with my own family. Yet during this relatively brief interval, I felt very insecure about my future. I am quite convinced that if I did not have tenure, I would have been dismissed from the job and institution that I loved. This feeling exaggerated and prolonged my stress and contributed to my sleeplessness, night sweats, nightmares, depression, moodiness, and a tendency to becoming angered and impatient. It also caused uneasy breathing bordering on panic attacks. Within several months of the incident, I required considerable dental repair, including crowns placed on several molars. My dentist attributed this to grinding my teeth during sleep. Many of these emotional manifestations resurfaced and became exacerbated whenever I met up with Dr. Starzl, even long after our professional interaction had ended.

Unquestionably, this experience tested my resolve and ability to tolerate stress; however, I believe that my character and resolve emerged largely unscathed and even strengthened by facing such adversity. Unfortunately, despite the passing of three decades, my heretofore high capacity to tolerate stress remains impaired. Thankfully, these post-traumatic stress-like disorder (PTSD) manifestations diminished as I approached retirement and my professional responsibilities decreased.

During this difficult period, numerous colleagues and other hospital personnel at CHP signed a petition indicating that my concerns and suggestions had merit and were fully justified. In addition, many former and current families under my care, expressed their unwavering love and support for me. They praised me for my integrity and for having the courage to defend my convictions, and for standing-up on behalf of my patients.

A letter that I found particularly helpful in boosting my morale was sent to me by Dr. Jack Reinhart, the psychologist who initially opposed renal transplantation in young children (see p. 26). He had relocated from Pittsburgh to Hendersonville, North Carolina, but somehow kept up with news at CHP. He wrote, "I hope you 'ill get the support you need from Dr. Oliver, Donaldson and the other faculty members who must know and understand your problem. And I just wanted you to know that I completely agree with you and admire your integrity."

Another heartwarming and very supportive letter came from my former chairman of pediatrics, Dr. Tim Oliver. In it he wrote, "It is hardly possible for me to thank you for all that you have done in developing a first-class Division of Pediatric Nephrology and for your expectations and demands for high quality behavior of peers. Despite the resentments, the joy of what has emerged is your honesty, commitment and integrity. I've known that longer than anyone in the School-Department. You have my unwavering respect and affection."

Unbeknown to me at the time, the circumstances of my crisis were closely monitored by the broader University of Pittsburgh faculty. A letter that represented the wide support I received from this community was written by Dr. Robert Glew from the School of Biochemistry, whom I only knew peripherally. He wrote, "I applaud your courage in defending the welfare and interests of your patients. You honor medicine and the University of Pittsburgh School of Medicine when you defend your principles and the high standards of integrity we expect of the profession. I know you must be suffering; but take hart for you will be remembered for the generous and difficult thing you have done in challenging irresponsibility, egoism and accountability. Your actions have won the admiration of many. Keep the faith and good luck with your work."

I do not know to what extent, if any, this crisis served as a catalyst for the recruitment in July 1, 1987, of Dr. Richard Simmons-an internationally acclaimed chief of adult and pediatric transplantation at the University of Minnesota. He assumed the position of Chairman of the Department of Surgery at the University of Pittsburgh, School of Medicine. Through meetings with many members of the surgical staff who shared my concerns, Dr. Simmons had become very familiar with the issues raised in my memorandum. More importantly, as Dr. Starzl's de facto boss, he was not only empowered but had no reservation in implementing my suggestions.

To accomplish this, our pediatric renal transplant program had to be free of interference by Dr. Starzl and not be encumbered from the existing strained interpersonal relations. Given Dr. Simmons extensive pediatric transplant experience, our jointly devised diplomatic plan called for him to personally take charge of this particular program. We then agreed to assign two outstanding, locally trained young surgeons to perform the renal transplants at CHP under the supervision of Dr. Simmons. Both Drs. R. Shapiro and V. Scantlebury were most excited at the opportunity to function more independently and work with me to resolve the above transplant issues, including performing living donor kidney transplants in close collaboration and involvement of me and my staff. Both were highly intelligent and possessed great energy and outstanding surgical and interpersonal skills. They were also amenable to cooperating with our pediatric urologists in transplanting children with urologic disorders. Together, we formulated CHP's overall pediatric renal transplant management strategy. After lowering the goal blood cyclosporine level and refining our immunosuppressive protocol we achieved a marked improvement in kidney survival and had vastly fewer complications. In addition, we established combined daily renal and surgical transplant ward rounds, a dedicated pediatric renal transplant clinic, and a weekly renal transplant conference to review our experiences and ensure ongoing quality of care. This team effort fostered much mutual respect and the ensuing harmony between physicians and nurses had a very positive influence on patient care and gave much comfort to their families.

In 1989 we replaced cyclosporine with FK-506, a novel immunosuppressive agent (later renamed tacrolimus or Prograf). Our unique and simple regimen consisting only of tacrolimus and limited use of steroids, enabled us to achieve the best renal transplant outcomes in the world (100% for the first year after transplantation, Ellis D, et al: *Current expectations in pediatric renal transplantation. Current Opin in Organ Transplant 1:37-43, 1996*). Among these patients was the apprehensive-looking ten-month-old boy, pictured with me on the book cover in my secondary role as surrogate parent. I was trying to distract him and soothe his abdominal discomfort three days after transplantation. The kidney he received from his mother together with this immunosuppressive regimen served him well for over twenty-two years. Our protocol also enabled preadolescent children to resume growth and achieve a final height that surpassed all prior expectations. These notable successes evolving in large part out of my stand on behalf of my patients against "Goliath", served as reminders that my sacrifice was worthwhile. These achievements also boosted my sense of pride and joy, thereby palliating the lingering pain ushered by my crisis.

In closing this section of the book, I wish to underscore that as much as my personal opinions on immunosuppressive and other management issues conflicted with those of Dr. Starzl and were responsible for my most painful professional crisis, I also acknowledge and respect his many and noteworthy accomplishments. Undoubtedly, numerous organ recipients are alive today largely because of his surgical competence and tireless devotion to his craft. However, I do think that his inflexibility in adopting a less toxic, yet effective cyclosporine-based immunosuppressive regimen is a significant blemish to his great legacy.

Fortunately, over the past two decades, medical schools have become less oligarchical and encourage transparency and discourse in resolving health care-related concerns. Moreover, they have adopted a more conciliatory, rather than a polarizing, attitude toward their employees. These measures not only lead to better patient care but also benefit physicians and universities alike.

Demetri the philosopher?

Just because I am proud of my Greek heritage, I do not flatter or delude myself that I possess a gift for philosophical thinking. I must hasten to add, however, that in my experience, many of my modern Greek acquaintances, even those without much formal education, demonstrate an aptitude and enthusiasm for philosophical discourse. Perhaps this is most obvious at informal gatherings and outdoor cafés throughout Greece, where political ideas are debated with passion only rivaled by the passion they have for soccer. Most Greeks are keenly aware of how philosophy governs the principles that we apply in our daily lives. On many occasions throughout my life, I have examined my own objectivity and fairness and considered the importance of trust, respect, commitment, and love. Admittedly, on some occasions, I have also questioned a few doctrines of my Greek Orthodox religion. I have wondered if a change in the definition or concept of religion can be universally accepted to deter violence and senseless conflicts. A simple, nondenominational, and perhaps somewhat naive description of religion that I subscribe to is: Religion is that inner voice that reminds one to give comfort and help to the needy in all walks of life who, like myself, respect the laws of nature and live in peace and harmony with their fellow man.

Personally, I make no distinction between philosophy that is formally taught at institutions of higher learning and philosophy that is expressed in simple, colorful quotations. In addition, I see no reason for defining a "philosophical quotation" as one that is attributed solely to a classical or modern philosopher. Regardless of their origin, adherence to concepts captured in philosophical phrases can have a powerful impact in shaping one's way of life and inspiring one to behave in a constructive manner. Several of the ancient Greeks, such as Plato and Aristotle, elevated philosophy into a formal course of study that intrigued and inspired the greatest human minds. Their philosophical thinking encompassed abstract ideas and metaphysical concepts such as the existence of the soul, the meaning of life, and man's place in the universe. Their ideas laid the foundation of democracy as we know it today. The evolution of humans over the centuries has opened new areas of contemplation that have had profound influence on politics, science, and how one views our modern word. Recent themes that provoke philosophical thinking range from violations of basic human rights, a woman's right to abortion and influence of religion, moral and ethical issues surrounding euthanasia, proliferation and ownership of weapons of mass destruction and the potential destruction of humankind, why or who should regulate technology as to protect and individual's right to privacy, the societal effects of disparities in education and wealth, etc. Perhaps deserving greater contemplation and debate are the moral and ethical implications emanating from the genetic revolution, including the huge implications emanating from potential for unauthorized use of personal genetic information, genetic editing and genetic modification of plants, stem cells, embryos and animals, etc. These topics are well outside the scope of this book or my expertise. However, important challenges tended to focus my attention on certain perhaps more mundane philosophical themes. Below I offer some insight on *humility*.

As noted in the anecdote *"Bobby's sad predicament— a paradigm of raw courage and resolve"* (p. 79 and again in recounting Mamas story in *Medical malpractice suits: anathema for physicians* (p. 168), I experienced immense helplessness or ineptitude, both personally and professionally. It was as if all my efforts to acquire medical knowledge and skills were suddenly rendered useless; I simply felt defeated and small by the problems I was facing. These circumstances caused me to question the meaning and influence of *humility* on human behavior. I conclude that by allowing me to accept my limitations, humility enabled me to forgive myself and counteracted my negative emotions. in addition to promoting honesty in all interactions, humility strengthens many positive traits, such as listening, respecting and having empathy for others. Genuine humility is a strong impetus for constructive and positive thinking that can stimulate one's efforts towards perfecting their craft and ultimately gaining fulfillment. In contrast, I believe that false or contrived humility is the worst form of hypocrisy and is very counterproductive.

There are several clues that can help identify an individual who displays false humility. One is that he/she goes to great lengths to demonstrate their "humility" publicly. In fact, humble people tend to avoid media exposure. Another clue is promising unrealistic outcomes or unachievable goals. Yet other important clues are the intentional use of a soft voice, excessive expression of sympathy and the use of hand gestures to convey concepts that they alone seem to be able to grasp.

For as long as I can remember, I have used pertinent quotations to enhance my lectures and talks. My interest in reading and recollecting philosophical quotations began early in my childhood. I recall being mystified and intrigued when, as a young child, I came across one of Plato's assays on euthanasia in a college textbook on Greek philosophy belonging to an uncle of mine. It was written in ancient rather than modern Greek. My uncle attempted to explain it to me, but it was too challenging for a fourth grader. After all, this paragraph took scholars volumes of books to analyze over the next two millennia. Portions of Plato's insightful perspective on euthanasia is still pertinent to the modern-day debate on active -as in assisted suicide, and passive euthanasia. Ever since, the idea of distilling an important human trait or concept of nature into as few words as possible has greatly appealed to me. In my opinion, the ancient Greek language and philosophical tradition is especially suitable for this. However, at the risk of incurring the wrath of Hippocrates, Asklepios, or other of my Greek physician progenitors, I would like to mention a few of these non-Greek quotations that have some relevance to medicine:

"Diagnosis is one of the commonest diseases." —Karl Christian Krause, German philosopher

"If you are once in the habit of guessing, you are diagnostically drained." —Sir Robert Hutchison

"Irrationally held truths may be more harmful than reasoned errors." —Thomas Huxley, English biologist who strongly supported Charles Darwin's theories

"What we call experience is often a dreadful list of ghastly mistakes." —Chalmers Da Costa, surgeon in nineteenth century

"If you are not thinking what you are doing, then you are doing what you are thinking?" —Yogi Berra

"Thus, I saw that most men only care for science so far as they get a living from it, and they worship even error when it affords them sustenance." —Jonathan Wolfgang Goethe (This quotation may be used to justify why some physicians involved in academic medicine may resort to plagiarism to advance and sustain their careers).

"Science is the topography of ignorance. The best part of our knowledge is that which teaches us where knowledge leaves off and ignorance begins." —Oliver Wendell Holmes

"Science is a first-rate piece of furniture for a man's upper chamber, if he has common sense on the ground floor." —Oliver Wendell Holmes

"A physician who treats himself has a fool for a patient." —Sir William Osler

"The expert is seldom in doubt but frequently in error." —Unknown

"For a person of modest talent, modesty is the truth; for a person of great talent, modesty is hypocrisy." —Unknown

"We know the truth not only by reason but by the heart." —Blaise Pascal

"The truth cleverly told may be the biggest lie of all." —Thomas Hardy

"The heart is wiser than the intellect." —Unknown

"The biggest tragedy of life is not death but what dies within us while we live." —Unknown

"The bee that sucks the honey from the flower also pollinates it." —Unknown

"When darkness is thickest, you see the stars better." —Unknown

"When you get out on the road, you face many detours. Unless you know where you are going, you will never get there." —Mahatma Gandhi

Aptitude + Attitude = Altitude —Lionel Richie's father on equation for success

"A mind, like a parachute, does not work until open." —Charlie Chan episode in which Charlie gives advice to his son

"Medicine has not only given me a career but also the joy of doing my life's work." —Demetri Ellis

"I owe a great debt of gratitude to my parents, who taught me how to live a rich life without actually being rich." —Demetri Ellis

"Do not judge what others do by what you do but do the best job in whatever you do." —Demetri Ellis

"Medical knowledge is in constant flux, but the doctor-patient relationship endures and may make the difference between the will to live or die." —Demetri Ellis

"When you are about to make an important (medical) decision, stop and think for a moment; if you have any doubt or trepidation about the consequences of your actions, do not follow through! You will then arrive at the correct decision." —Demetri Ellis

"Even the soap dish needs to be washed from time to time." —Demetri Ellis

"The kidney is the soul of the body. The whole body is constructed to protect the kidneys." —combination of Jewish saying and Demetri Ellis' aggrandizement of the renal specialty

"The great variety of titles accorded to renal disorders is a tribute to the diversity of the kidney as an organ and a credit to the inventiveness and imagination of nephrologists." —Demetri Ellis

"The kidney epitomizes form and function." —Demetri Ellis

"While both the brain and kidney are regarded as pragmatic organs that enable one to adapt effectively to their environment, only the kidney behaves rationally." —Demetri Ellis

"Good judgment is based on experience and experience is based on poor judgment." —Demetri Ellis

"To write prescriptions is easy; to come to an understanding with patients is hard." —Franz Kafka

Cogito ergo sum." (I think, therefore I am) —Rene Descartes, as proof of his existence

Edo ergo sum." (I eat, therefore I am) — Unknown

"It is not enough to have a good mind; the main thing is to use it." —Rene Descartes

"The greatest minds are capable of the greatest vices as well as the greatest virtues." —Rene Descartes

"A horse is a camel designed by committee." —Unknown

"A meeting is an organized way of prolonging decisions or justifying one's job." —Unknown

"If you cannot convince them, confuse them." —President Harry Truman

"My memory is like a policeman; I cannot find it when I need it." —Anonymous

HIPPOCRARES, ASKLEPIOS, AND DEMETRI ELLIS?
HISTORICAL PERSPECTIVE OF MY CAREER

As a person of Greek heritage, it would be inappropriate and possibly sacrilegious of me not to mention some of my ancestors who laid the foundation for the practice of medicine as we know it today. It would also be presumptuous, if not laughable or even absurd, for me to mention my name in the same sentence as my famous ancestors. However, in the same vein that inspired the ancient Greeks, I also share the need, if not the gift, to engage in philosophical discourse.

All modern physicians, as well as many laymen, are familiar with the Hippocratic Oath (see below), written by Hippocrates, "the father of medicine," in the third century BCE. Hippocrates was undoubtedly influenced by the teachings of the followers of Asklepios over the previous two centuries. In fact, the original Hippocratic Oath began by, "I swear by Apollo the Physician and by Asklepios and by Hygieia and Panacea and by all the gods." Asklepios was the god of medicine. According to ancient Greek religion, he was one of Apollo's sons, sharing with Apollo the epithet *Paean* ("the Healer"). Apollo carried Asklepios as a baby to the centaur Chiron who raised Asklepios and instructed him in the art of medicine. It is said that in return for the kindness rendered by Asklepios, a snake licked Asklepios's ears clean and imbued him with medical secrets (to the ancient Greeks snakes were sacred beings of wisdom, healing, and resurrection). Asklepios is often depicted with a rod entwined with a snake, which to this day remains the symbol of medicine/the art of healing. In fact, the healing temples or Asklepieia are the forerunners of today's hospitals.

From its inception, modern medicine as envisaged by the doctrines of Asklepios and Hippocrates was a unique profession based on a covenant of trust between the healer and the afflicted. According to current opinion, to effectively dispense his/her responsibilities, a physician must possess the qualities of "humility, honesty, intellectual integrity, compassion, and effacement of excessive self-interest." Physicians have the fiduciary duty to place the interest of patients above their own. It is widely believed that that this relationship has been significantly compromised in the era of managed care. (Christine K. Cassel, M.D. The Patient-Physician Covenant: An Affirmation of Asklepios. *Ann. Intern. Med.* 1996;124(6):604-606. Crawshaw R., Rogers D.E., Pellegrino E.D., Bulger R.J., Lundberg G.D., Bristow L.R., *et al.* Patient-physician covenant. *JAMA.* 1995; 273:1553. Bailey J.E. Asklepios: ancient hero of medical caring. *Ann. Intern. Med.* 1996; 124:257-63.)

Below are an original Greek version and an English translation of the Hippocratic Oath:

ΟΡΚΟΣ

Ὄμνυμι Ἀπόλλωνα ἰητρὸν καὶ Ἀσκληπιὸν
καὶ Ὑγείαν καὶ Πανάκειαν καὶ θεοὺς πάντας τε
καὶ πάσας, ἵστορας ποιεύμενος, ἐπιτελέα ποιήσειν
κατὰ δύναμιν καὶ κρίσιν ἐμὴν ὅρκον τόνδε καὶ
συγγραφὴν τήνδε· ἡγήσεσθαι μὲν τὸν διδάξαντά
με τὴν τέχνην ταύτην ἴσα γενέτῃσιν ἐμοῖς,
καὶ βίου κοινώσεσθαι, καὶ χρεῶν χρηίζοντι
μετάδοσιν ποιήσεσθαι, καὶ γένος τὸ ἐξ αὐτοῦ
ἀδελφοῖς ἴσον ἐπικρινεῖν ἄρρεσι, καὶ διδάξειν
10 τὴν τέχνην ταύτην, ἢν χρηίζωσι μανθάνειν, ἄνευ
μισθοῦ καὶ συγγραφῆς, παραγγελίης τε καὶ
ἀκροήσιος καὶ τῆς λοίπης ἁπάσης μαθήσιος
μετάδοσιν ποιήσεσθαι υἱοῖς τε ἐμοῖς καὶ τοῖς τοῦ
ἐμὲ διδάξαντος, καὶ μαθητῇσι συγγεγραμμένοις
τε καὶ ὡρκισμένοις νόμῳ ἰητρικῷ, ἄλλῳ δὲ οὐδενί.
διαιτήμασί τε χρήσομαι ἐπ᾽ ὠφελείῃ καμνόντων
κατὰ δύναμιν καὶ κρίσιν ἐμήν, ἐπὶ δηλήσει δὲ
καὶ ἀδικίῃ εἴρξειν. οὐ δώσω δὲ οὐδὲ φάρμακον
οὐδενὶ αἰτηθεὶς θανάσιμον, οὐδὲ ὑφηγήσομαι συμ-
20 βουλίην τοιήνδε· ὁμοίως δὲ οὐδὲ γυναικὶ πεσσὸν
φθόριον δώσω. ἁγνῶς δὲ καὶ ὁσίως διατηρήσω
βίον τὸν ἐμὸν καὶ τέχνην τὴν ἐμήν. οὐ τεμέω
δὲ οὐδὲ μὴν λιθιῶντας,[1] ἐκχωρήσω δὲ ἐργάτῃσιν

ἀνδράσι πρήξιος τῆσδε. ἐς οἰκίας δὲ ὁκόσας ἂν
ἐσίω, ἐσελεύσομαι ἐπ᾽ ὠφελείῃ καμνόντων, ἐκτὸς
ἐὼν πάσης ἀδικίης ἑκουσίης καὶ φθορίης, τῆς τε
ἄλλης καὶ ἀφροδισίων ἔργων ἐπί τε γυναικείων
σωμάτων καὶ ἀνδρῴων, ἐλευθέρων τε καὶ δούλων.
ἃ δ᾽ ἂν ἐν θεραπείῃ ἢ ἴδω ἢ ἀκούσω, ἢ καὶ ἄνευ
30 θεραπείης κατὰ βίον ἀνθρώπων, ἃ μὴ χρή ποτε
ἐκλαλεῖσθαι ἔξω, σιγήσομαι, ἄρρητα ἡγεύμενος
εἶναι τὰ τοιαῦτα. ὅρκον μὲν οὖν μοι τόνδε ἐπιτελέα ποιέοντι, καὶ μὴ συγχέοντι, εἴη ἐπαύρασθαι
καὶ βίου καὶ τέχνης δοξαζομένῳ παρὰ πᾶσιν
ἀνθρώποις ἐς τὸν αἰεὶ χρόνον· παραβαίνοντι δὲ
36 καὶ ἐπιορκέοντι, τἀναντία τούτων.

[1] Littré suggests αἰτέοντας, Reinhold οὐδὲ μὴ ἐν ἡλικίῃ ἐόντας.

OATH

I swear by Apollo Physician, by Asclepius, by Health, by Panacea and by all the gods and goddesses, making them my witnesses, that I will carry out, according to my ability and judgment, this oath and this indenture. To hold my teacher in this art equal to my own parents; to make him partner in my livelihood; when he is in need of money to share mine with him; to consider his family as my own brothers, and to teach them this art, if they want to learn it, without fee or indenture; to impart precept,[1] oral instruction, and all other instruction[2] to my own sons, the sons of my teacher, and to indentured pupils who have taken the physician's oath, but to nobody else. I will use treatment to help the sick according to my ability and judgment, but never with a view to injury and wrong-doing. Neither will I administer a poison to anybody when asked to do so, nor will I suggest such a course. Similarly I will not give to a woman a pessary to cause abortion. But I will keep pure and holy both my life and my art. I will not use the knife, not even, verily, on sufferers from stone, but I will give place to such as are craftsmen therein. Into whatsoever houses I enter, I will enter to help the sick, and I will abstain from all intentional wrong-doing and harm, especially from abusing the bodies of man or woman, bond or free. And whatsoever I shall see or hear in the course of my profession, as well as outside my profession in my intercourse with men,[2] if it be what should not be published abroad, I will never divulge, holding such things to be holy secrets. Now if I carry out this oath, and break it not, may I gain for ever reputation among all men for my life and for my art; but if I transgress it and forswear myself, may the opposite befall me.

[1] Apparently the written rules of the art, examples of which are to be found in several Hippocratic treatises. These books were not published in the strict sense of the word, but copies would be circulated among the members of the "physicians' union."
[2] Probably, in modern English, "instruction, written, oral and practical."

299

[2] This remarkable addition is worthy of a passing notice. The physician must not gossip, no matter how or where the subject-matter for gossip may have been acquired; whether it be in practice or in private life makes no difference.

In concluding this section, I urge the reader to read further and discover my philosophical views on what constitutes an outstanding physician. I believe that such appraisal requires experience and perspective, that I hope is evident in my *Advice to my residents and fellows*.

ADVICE TO MY RESIDENTS AND FELLOWS: STRIVE TO BE THE BEST!

———❧———

PHYSICIANS FORMULATE THEIR own criteria that define an exceptional doctor. Common attributes include certain innate traits such as a charismatic personality that facilitates interpersonal engagement and empathy, a handsome appearance, wit, humor, and a variety of other interpersonal skills. Additionally, having a superb professional reputation among their peers is an essential element. Many of us have admired such virtues in a few select former teachers and mentors who have contributed to our personal development. Other important qualities, however, may be underappreciated because they are less obvious and, in some cases, more subjective. Many of these tend to emerge out of one's experiences with unique patients who had a profound influence in shaping a physician's approach in delivering medical care. As my personal medical experience and knowledge expanded, I began to develop my own standards of medical excellence. A compilation of these standards constitutes my *Advice to my residents and fellows: Strive to be the best!* These tenets or principles may be especially valuable to students, physicians in training programs, and younger faculty. They may also aid patients and families in selecting a personal physician who embodies these principles. Of greatest benefit to patients is the selection of physicians who remain "competent" and provide care based on the most current scientific data (*see, Medical competence is paramount for physicians and patients*). For physicians caring for patients with chronic disorders, sometimes over decades, such as myself, I consider "*Bonding well with patients and families ...*" as being equally important. This engagement is essential for attaining better disease outcomes and ultimately is a key source of work satisfaction and joy in doctor's lives. This explains why I elect to begin by first discussing this tenet. The order of importance or priority of the other principles is somewhat arbitrary.

BONDING WELL WITH FAMILIES AND CHILDREN IS THE KEY TO DISEASE OUTCOME

Throughout my career I derived much satisfaction from my academic accomplishments. However, I most enjoyed and valued the strong personal connections I cultivated with my patients and their families. Such engagement was essential for achieving the foremost objective of medical care, improving the disease outcome of the child. As noted below, however, this was also of profound benefit to me. From a pragmatic standpoint, strong bonds with families also reduce the chances for medical malpractice suits as well as translate into significant financial support of both clinical and basic research, as I related earlier in the book. Hence, it is worth reminding younger physicians to balance time devoted to tabulating patient data in the electronic medical record with time invested in establishing genuine personal connections with families. As noted in the section titled, *The changing face of the medical profession* (see p. 222), the inability of currently practicing physicians to devote sufficient time to this latter task is a key factor limiting physician satisfaction.

I utilized several important approaches in establishing a strong personal bond right from my initial interaction with families. Because this endeavor can be very time consuming, I again resorted to my toolbox of optimizing the use of time, as described in *Demetri: a model of efficiency*, in p. 45. Thus, I devised a thorough Medical History

Questionnaire that the family completed just prior to our clinic interaction. This information complemented my prior review of requested medical records. The fact that I was well informed and prepared to address the child's medical condition quickly yet comprehensively was very reassuring to the families.

Realizing that children do not live in isolation and rely on their parents for health care and other decisions that influence their lives, my most important next step consisted of connecting with children and their families on a personal level thereby earning their respect. This demands actions and not just words on the part of the physician. Certain family lifestyles can be challenging for doctors to address but taking an adversarial or criticizing attitude may end up undermining the care of the child. At the same time, as a pediatrician, I leave no doubt that the interests of the child always supersede those of their family; my priority is to be the child's advocate and deliver the best care possible. Thus, it is essential to convince the child and their family that you are their advocate and you genuinely care for them, that you are committed to making their medical fight your own fight as well. As an example, I occasionally came to the CHP ED to see a child after regular work hours and offered my apologies for being dressed in athletic gear and sweaty. However, without exception, the families were understanding and appreciated that I had come to attend to them promptly and in person. This nearly always fostered respect from the family.

It is important to keep in mind that earning the family's trust and respect is often a slow process that requires the application of several key components. First, remember to be a good listener and listen with the intent to learn and not just wait for your chance to respond. Remind yourself of the Buddhist proverb, "If your mouth is open, you are not learning" and that even teachers and preachers need to listen. In addition, observe the patient's body language for cues that give greater context to what they say. For instance, during a family history review I was informed that the child's father had recently hanged themselves and everyone became tearful at recalling this event. Clearly, a time out was needed to express sympathy rather than proceed with the next question. Learn of the family's concerns but reserve your judgment until you have gathered all the necessary information. Then, you must clearly explain what you think is wrong with the child (differential diagnosis), how you plan to evaluate the condition, explain how serious it is, spell out in detail your management plan, discuss what metrics (test results or markers) you plan to use as evidence of improvement, and conclude with an estimate of the ultimate prognosis. All this must be communicated using language that the child and parent can clearly understand. Physicians must be aware that by overwhelming the family with excessive medical information, they may be perceived as arrogant and thus undermine the partnership approach to optimal clinical outcomes.

I must confess that during the earlier part of my career, on extremely rare occasion, if the child had an incurable genetic diagnosis, I advised against divulging the poor prognosis to the child. This practice may be questionable from a legal standpoint, but in my opinion, it was justified. I reasoned that it was not in the best interest of the child to live with the constant fear of their disease long before they actually became symptomatic. Being fully aware of the eventually poor prognosis can cause profound psychological trauma; a fatalistic attitude can alter a child's perception of their future, thereby impairing their intellectual growth and development. Someone recently coined the term *previvor*, rather than *survivor*, to describe individuals living with an incurable or progressive illness.

The importance of building strong personal connections with the children and families under my care became quite evident very early during my career in Pittsburgh. I soon realized that there was no support group for families with children affected by chronic renal disorders. In my view, for such an organization to succeed, it had to be a parent-led endeavor. Support groups were not easy to set up in the years prior to the internet, email, and social media apps. Families had to be individually contacted by telephone or regular mail. With my encouragement, several industrious parents collaborated with me to establish the first Renal Parent Support Group. As their inaugural event, they planned a very enjoyable picnic at Fox Chapel Park in Pittsburgh in 1980. There, I introduced the families to other families in the same predicament. They realized they were not alone and were particularly impressed by the healthy appearance and level of physical activity of children with kidney transplants. This gave much comfort and hope to other families whose children were prospective transplant recipients. The photo below shows the participants at that picnic. My family attended as well, sending a message of solidarity.

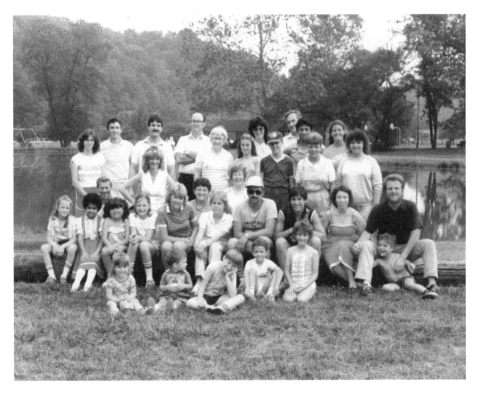

The picnic was a huge success and the Renal Parent Support Group flourished and became permanent. Each subsequent year, we organized a Christmas Party, a Renal Kids Summer Camp and a Walkathon. As the number of participants grew much larger, these events were underwritten by the Pittsburgh Chapter of the National Kidney Foundation of Western PA that was established in 1982. I also informally discussed several renal topics of common interest to families and others willing to attend these conferences on late evenings.

Having a deep and caring renal staff was also instrumental in developing closer relationships with our patients and their families. In my view, this team effort was a key ingredient of our recipe for successful disease outcomes. This connection evolved to the point that many patients and their families regarded our nephrology staff as family. We intentionally cultivated this surrogate-relative role by sending greeting cards to celebrate the child's milestones. We also actively encouraged many patients to pursue a college education; I wrote many recommendation letters on their behalf and followed their educational progress with great pride and joy.

MEDICAL COMPETENCE IS PARAMOUNT
FOR PHYSICIANS AND PATIENTS

While physician competence is essential for improving disease outcomes, this key attribute may be difficult to discern. Thus, I caution patients and their families, "don't judge a book by its cover". Although all physicians wish to be perceived as knowledgeable, it may be challenging for themselves and for their patients to ascertain where a physician fits in the spectrum of competence. A trusted primary care provider may be the best source of information in selecting a reputable specialist but word-of-mouth from friends or relatives or an interrogation of multiple internet resources, may also aid this important process.

Attaining and sustaining competence requires much effort and a high degree of motivation driven by the fundamental concept that advances in science offer the exciting prospect of discovering answers to disease mechanisms and inventing novel, more effective therapies. To become competent, one must be systematic, determined, and passionate about his/her work. For me, attaining competence started by making the effort to master the basic sciences and clinical aspects of pediatrics and nephrology. However, maintaining competence was an ongoing and far more challenging objective. Fortunately, the kidney was always interesting, enigmatic and even magical to me, making me a student for life. From the beginning of my career, I developed an outline of my scientific article filing system, which greatly aided the systematic filing and retrieval of important scientific articles well before the availability of computers and the internet, which eventually made this task much less tedious. I read these articles carefully, underlined important passages, ranked their importance based on the quality of the evidence presented, special notes were often added on the front page, and, finally, I signed them. The latter was important because it encouraged those who borrowed these articles to return the original copy back to me.

To help assess and reinforce one's perception of competence in managing serious medical conditions, one must adhere to succinct yet detailed documentation and periodic objective review of the clinical data. Ultimately, the data must be analyzed and published in reputable journals. The latter is essential for confirming the validity of the results and for eventually developing a consensus opinion among the experts on the most effective treatment plan for any given disorder. To enable me to accomplish these tasks, I brought this sort of work with me everywhere, even during brief vacations with my family. Receiving favorable reviews of my work from esteemed journal editors and colleagues and witnessing management trends that I pioneered become the standard of care both nationally and internationally gave me a great deal of satisfaction and intensified my resolve to remain current in my field. As a result, my love for nephrology has grown with the passing of time. While the nephrology specialty is demanding, challenging, and time-consuming, I feel very fortunate to be doing what I love for a living.

FOCUS ON PATHOMECHANISMS OF DISEASE

My current files contain tens of thousands of articles that attest to the time I invested in developing a strong foundation for my work;

this wealth of information helped me to think of diseases in terms of their mechanisms, or *pathophysiology*. I reasoned that if I could comprehend normal physiology, I could better appreciate pathophysiology. The better I understood the pathophysiology of a disorder, the more confident I became in designing a scientific, fact-based and potentially more effective management plan. In fact, I have repeatedly discovered that any intervention that interferes with normal or adaptive physiologic or homeostatic mechanisms is more likely to harm rather than help an individual. Conversely, interventions that interrupt pathophysiologic processes increase the odds of recovery. During my career, I have repeatedly demonstrated to my residents and fellows the advantages of applying this paradigm in the evaluation and management of children with complex medical disorders. A good example of the practical application of this concept is in the management of edema—body swelling—in children with nephrotic syndrome (see, Ellis, D. Pathophysiology, Evaluation, and Management of Edema in Childhood Nephrotic Syndrome. Front. Pediatr., 11 January 2016 | https://doi.org/10.3389/fped.2015.00111).

BUILT BRIDGES AND PROMOTE COLLABORATION

During my long pediatric nephrology career, I managed numerous children with complex and very challenging disorders. Getting the best outcome in such individuals often requires a great deal of professional collaboration. I like to think that one of my personal strengths is to engage pathologists, bacteriologists, ICU staff, nurses, social workers, dieticians, behavioral psychologists, pharmacists, and other talented colleagues that can contribute to the care of my patients. While we did not always agree, we always respected each other's opinion. Building strong bridges and enlisting such cooperative effort was invaluable in achieving optimal patient care. Concurrently, co-authorship of articles describing good disease outcomes in various journals served our personal career objectives as well. This strong spirit of collaboration inevitably led to excellent renal transplant and other disease outcomes at CHP, even at times when human and financial resources were limited.

INFORM FAMILIES OF THE RISKS AND BENEFITS OF MEDICAL INTERVENTIONS, BUT TAKE DECISIVE ACTION

I have always made a conscious effort to refrain from using new therapies that tend to expose children to unreasonable risks or potential harm. However, faced with challenging or seemingly insurmountable medical disorders, I made a strong effort to devise innovative therapies. If the proposed regimen had scientific underpinnings supporting potential benefits and those exceeded the risks, I was comfortable in offering such options to families. I found the following line in "An Essay on Criticism" by Alexander Pope, to be a useful reminder when applying this principle in making decisions throughout my career:

"Be not the first by whom the new are tried,
Nor yet the last to lay the old aside."

ACT IN A TIMELY MANNER

Throughout my career, I welcomed being contacted at any time of the day to contribute my input on a management plan rather than find fault with a treatment plan that had been already implemented to the detriment of the patient. This obviates the need for damage control measures, including transferring blame to someone else or making excuses to the children and their families after an avoidable mishap. Applying sound and consistent management decisions on a timely manner led to faster recovery from an illness and enabled the systematic assessment of outcomes of specific disorders. This approach also enhanced my confidence in making medical decisions. Successful outcomes also validated my efforts and gave me the resolve to endure long working hours without any regrets.

AVOID OVER-TESTING OR OVER-PRESCRIBING MEDICATIONS

Performing the fewest procedures necessary to effectively diagnose and manage a medical condition best serves the interests of the patient. Limiting the number and dosages of prescribed medications is equally important. Application of these caveats helps curb the cost of medical care; more importantly, however, these measures help reduce or avoid potential complications and adverse effects of procedures and medications that may then result in even more interventions. Practicing this philosophy—being a reductionist or minimalist—is one of the fundamental principles that force a doctor to think deliberately and systematically. Implied in this concept is that a physician will not be deterred from applying any interventions if they are medically indicated. In my experience, expressing this concept to children and their families is very reassuring to them because it indicates that you share their concerns and that you have their best interests in mind. Such transparency was much appreciated by my patients and facilitated their commitment to the treatment plan, which is crucial in achieving desired disease outcomes. I believe that this concept is currently emphasized in many medical school and residency curricula.

ENCOURAGE ACTIVE PARENTAL INVOLVEMENT

I have always regarded children and their parents not only as capable, but also as necessary collaborators in our common purpose of improving the children's health. Therefore, I would typically outline a child's initial markers of disease activity and reviewed these with the families during follow-up clinic visits. I praised parents who could recall these markers from one visit to the next and based on such feedback I was convinced that they were fully invested in their child's health. An integral part of this process was to inform the families of potential adverse effects of medications and how to monitor for these, as well as what markers will be used to gauge the efficacy of any therapeutic intervention more objectively. Simultaneously, I emphasized that safety was the overriding priority. This reassured the family that, if needed, their medical regimen could and would be modified. In fact, such transparency facilitated all medical decisions. As discussed in an earlier section of this book (p. 168), the importance of transparency and admission of mistakes in deterring malpractice suits, cannot be understated.

BE HONEST AND ADMIT YOUR LIMITATIONS

As much time as we physicians may devote to understanding medicine and as much as our patients look upon us to have all the answers to their problems, we must accept the fact that we do not have and will likely never have all the answers. However, if we make a sincere effort to research the literature and seek advice from other colleagues on patients with complex disorders—i.e. leaving no stone unturned— we will have fulfilled the most important element of our patient-physician contract. Nearly all patients are willing to accept and even appreciate our admission of ignorance in dealing with challenging medical issues, so we need not fear that we will be perceived as inept. It is worth re-emphasizing that honesty and humility must be actively cultivated and liberally utilized while practicing medicine.

BALANCE THE ART AND SCIENCE OF MEDICINE

While the science of medicine tends to be quantifiable and well defined by the proof of principle rule, the art of medicine is more subjective. To me, these terms are complementary. Thus, a measure of both is necessary for physicians to be effective in practicing their craft. I believe the quote below from my respected colleague Dr. Sara McIntyre echoes my impressions of what constitutes an exceptional physician:

> "All conscientious physicians should make every effort to learn basic sciences and keep up with medical resources needed to maintain expertise in their field of interest. However, application of such information to the maximum benefit of the patient depends on "the art of medicine." This craft is gleaned from observing other colleagues whose medical skills we admire and respect, and whose manner we strive to emulate. The craft of "the art of medicine" is not something

you learn at school or at any given time, but rather it is an ongoing process that you must cultivate and nourish constantly and build from one's experience. It requires the physician to relate well and gain the trust and respect of people of all walks of life. The art comprises asking probing questions, listening well to the answers, demonstrating empathy, sincerity and genuine interest for the patient, and generating careful and sensible diagnostic and treatment plans that are appropriate and realistic for the individual patient under his/her care. Ultimately, the clear communication of the information utilizing language that is well understood by the patient, serves as the cornerstone to the effective implementation and achievement of all management goals. While there is no substitute for experience, these skills should be taught and emphasized to young physicians so that they develop a constant awareness of their importance".

Parting salutation on graduating from our renal fellowship program

In closing this section, I would like to share a simple Greek salutation that is typically expressed at the completion at any level of academic achievement: *Eis anotera*. It means, "May you aspire to higher," with the added words *learning* or *education* being implied. It also implies that learning is a continuum. This is well depicted by a sculpture by Jonathan Barofsky located at the entrance to the campus of Carnegie Mellon University in Pittsburgh showing people of various ages ascending a long, slanted pole pointing towards the sky. Indeed, when it comes to education the sky is the limit and the path to knowledge is infinite.

https://n7.alamy.com/zooms/007fe5d1528847adb80f18f3fbd 2e0be/carnegie-mellon-university-is-home-to-walking-to-the-sky-a-stainless-e6h82k.jpg

THE CHANGING FACE
OF THE MEDICAL PROFESSION

OVER THE PAST fifty years, the enactment of landmark legislation and implementation of novel social policies led to fundamental changes in health care delivery in the United States. The effects of these measures on the traditional practice of medicine were swift and far-reaching. Perhaps an unintended consequence was that physicians, collectively, became increasingly dissatisfied and disillusioned with multiple facets of their profession. According to sequential physician satisfaction or wellness surveys recently summed-up by the Association of American Medical Colleges, only 6% of physicians currently in private practice report a positive morale and an increasing number consider a change in career or would not recommend this profession to promising students. While less than 15% of physicians in 1973 doubted entering the right career, this number rose to 50% in 1980 and 61% in 2016 (https:// physiciansfoundation.org/wp-content/uploads/2017/12/2014_ Physicians_Foundation_Biennial_Physician_Survey_Report. pdf;https://www.aamc.org/download/473344/data/annualaddressof-thephysicianworkforce.pdf; https://pdfs.semanticscholar.org/dd6b/4 b662c2dfafd1e839a8f1da8af713a4106ac.pdf). Hence, there is growing concern that the number of primary care physicians will diminish in the future (https://www.aamc.org/download/473344/data/

annualaddressofthephysicianworkforce.pdf). To address the scope and causes of burnout or emotional exhaustion, many centers are currently utilizing proprietary tools, such as the one devised by the Physician Wellness Academic Consortium (PWAC), to anonymously collect and analyze pertinent data (https://wellmd.**stanford**.edu/center1/survey.html). The intent is to utilize this information constructively to find solutions that not only reduce burnout but also improve professional satisfaction and fulfilment. As an example, a survey from Stanford identified sleep-related impairment as being a major determinant of burnout and subsequently devised strategies for attenuating this problem. Moreover, an increasing number of institutions are appointing *wellness officers* to help health care providers cope with depression and work-related stress.

Concurrent with the dissatisfaction and disillusionment of physicians, patient satisfaction surveys also indicate that many patients perceive that the amount and quality of their medical care is diminishing. One survey cites several studies indicating a strong link between physician satisfaction and quality of patient care (https://pdfs.semanticscholar.org/dd6b/4b662c2dfafd1e839a8f1da8af713a4106ac.pdf). Along these lines, one may deduce that dissatisfied physicians will be less motivated to put the effort needed to remain current with advancements in medicine.

Interestingly, although the cost of medical education has risen markedly while fees for service and inflation-adjusted income to primary care physicians have actually declined, salary reduction is not reported as a primary cause of physician dissatisfaction. Also, the number of work hours and overall responsibilities that plagued solo private practitioners in the past have generally diminished and are not a major source of discontent. Leading the causes of dissatisfaction in today's physicians are loss of autonomy in decisions involving setting their hours of work and particularly the volume of patients that maintenance health organizations (HMOs) require physicians to see. That number has increased by nearly 100% causing 81% of doctors to feel overextended, stressed and unable to accept new patients. Doctor's opinions also diverge in other important respects from those of entrepreneurial HMOs that impose the rules of health care delivery. As a result, physicians continue to experience roadblocks when attempting to prescribe a more effective or less toxic medication that is not on the list of less expensive medications approved by the HMO or, despite much effort and time, they failed to convince the front-line HMO representative to permit delaying the discharge from the hospital of a patient with special needs or unexpected complications rather than based on their diagnosis upon admission.

Apart from the encompassing effects of the above society-driven transformative changes in the health care delivery, additional factors contribute to low satisfaction among physicians. These include: a. Lack of support or respect from patients, colleagues or affiliated institutions; b. the large amount of time spent on cumbersome billing schemes; c. while technology has enhanced maintenance and sharing of "paperless medical records", the cost of this enterprise has been very underestimated and also significantly reduces the time available for physicians to interact and cultivate the ever so important mutual respect and trust with their patients; d. exorbitant litigation rewards have resulted in high malpractice insurance premiums and promoted the practice of defensive medicine at an increased expense to doctors and patients alike (see, *Medical malpractice suits: anathema to physicians*, p. 168). These trends are alarming and have combined to erode the doctor-patient interaction and undermine the ideals of the medical profession and the status of being a doctor. The net result is increased emotional stress, diminished morale, and less self-fulfillment and overall physician satisfaction.

In addition, on a societal level, many doctors lament the fact that health care has become so expensive, politicized and often inaccessible to the poor, and thereby not benefitting all members of society. As a nation, the U.S. currently spends nearly 20% of gross domestic product (GDP) on health—the highest among any country—while not achieving the best outcomes. Major contributors to the rapidly rising cost of medical care include expansion of Medicare in 1971 and capitation to hospitals based on diagnosis starting in 1983, administration of medical services by HMOs starting in 1985, and the addition of prescription drug coverage by Medicare in 2006 contributing to accelerated drug prices in recent years. Many patients cannot afford preventive care and incur large out-of-pocket expenses when they seek routine care at the emergency department where doctors unfamiliar with their medical and social history tend to order expensive and often unnecessary tests. The quality or effectiveness of care of individuals without assigned primary care physicians may be further compromised by lack of preventive and follow-up care. In short, the collective effects of these pervasive ailments ultimately translate into more expensive and yet less effective care, that disproportionately harms disadvantaged individuals.

Because provision of preventive and follow-up care to all members of our society is not only a national mandate but also makes good financial sense, we must act quickly to remedy the existing problems. On their part, doctors must accept the fact that their profession has reached a new scientific, ideological and administrative set-point that cannot and should not be fully reversed. Hence, their efforts should focus on restoring the basic time-honored features of the traditional practice of medicine while welcoming and incorporating newer concepts that inevitably arise by evolving progress in science and technology. HMOs should clearly understand that the current medical care model is not sustainable because it is increasingly less cost-effective and because both doctors and patients are dissatisfied with it. To change the existing model will require the adoption of a comprehensive national health policy and its implementation by private providers. There are several specific reforms that can entice future promising students to pursue a medical career as well as improve morale and fulfillment among currently practicing physicians as to enhance patient care. These include restoring to physicians greater control of their practice, respecting their judgment as to the number of patients they are required to see, providing fair compensation for services, and reducing red tape and paperwork so that they can allocate more time in direct patient care. Another major challenge is to contain the recent marked escalation of medication costs and limit medical malpractice awards. While these are practical solutions, achieving them will require much resolve from the public and healthcare leaders, as well as bipartisan effort of policymakers to overcome opposition from special interest groups including private health care purveyors and the pharmaceutical industry. These concerns are of great importance to physicians and must be urgently addressed to avert a bigger crisis in our health care delivery system.

In the meantime, I wish to reassure my physician colleagues that dissatisfaction with our profession need not be inevitable or permanent. As an antidote to the existing vexing issues, I urge doctors to and re-commit and embrace the enduring albeit somewhat idealistic concepts of traditional medicine. These are richly depicted in the anecdotes and stories I relate throughout the book and are the source of the great joy and fulfilment I experienced throughout my career. The tenets listed in my *Advice to my residents and fellows: Strive to be the best!* (see, p. 209) also emanate directly from this proposed "back to the future-like" direction for the medical profession. In essence, these concepts represent a road map enabling doctors to remain on a path that will ultimately revitalize themselves and in the process empower them to become more effective healers.

RETIREMENT

STARTING IN JULY 2012, I began to relinquish many of my administrative duties and then, one by one, my academic duties. As a result, Dr. Bates became the director of pediatric nephrology at CHP, while Dr. Moritz assumed the position of clinical director. These are very talented, extremely bright, and caring individuals. More importantly, they are bound by the same beliefs. Hence, I felt assured that the baby that I had helped birth and raise will remain in very capable hands and that the mission I had envisioned for the nephrology division would continue to guide the care of my patients well into the future. Perhaps my marching song, "Nephron Man", can give them strength and inspire them to carry out this difficult but meritorious task.

As the next step in the process toward retirement, I gradually divested myself of clinical duties. I began to work part-time, mainly consisting of low-risk outpatient clinic evaluations, including supervision of the Friday clinic in conjunction with our junior renal fellows. This gave me the opportunity to start these young, aspiring nephrologists on the road to higher achievement by serving as a role model for them and by passing on my philosophy regarding the "ideal" physician. I also emphasized to them the importance of several of my techniques and guidelines on how to bond with children and their families. Another major objective of my interaction with fellows was to share with them my experience and perspective on many disorders.

I was finally able to shed the beeper that had been the harbinger of so many emergencies and constant interruptions over the years and had enslaved me since the start of my medical career. I no longer had night call or weekend call duties. Despite having my salary cut in half overnight, these were good enough reasons to celebrate.

Because of my more leisurely work pace, I enjoyed seeing patients and teaching even more. My fellows were eager to learn and practice my beloved specialty. However, despite the less stressful yet mentally stimulating daily regimen made possible by my part-time nephrology position, I missed terribly the stimulating interactions that I had over the years with many pediatric residents.

Mostly, however, I missed attending the pediatric renal transplant clinic through which, as a key member of the transplant team, I had cared for children with many serious and often congenital renal disorders requiring dialysis and renal transplantation. The lives of these children, their families, and mine became tightly interwoven. Moreover, I stopped attending presentations of interesting and challenging patients at renal and general pediatric grand rounds, as well as during our own sign-out rounds in the nephrology division. Attendance at research conferences was also limited or stopped. I also gradually reduced my lecture assignments. Not having to attend administrative meetings, conferences on medical informatics, and completion of annual mandatory modules on subjects only tangentially related to medical practice, gave me added joy as well as relief. Although I found it increasingly more difficult, I continued to write scientific articles on a steady basis because I found the experience challenging and a means for me to remain current with the literature on topics of interest to me.

It was only after I fully retired that I stopped to think about what motivated me to work such long hours during my entire career. In retrospect, my work appetite was fueled primarily by my love and commitment to the kidney. In my view, the kidney is at once complex and simple; it epitomizes the concept of *form and function* in its anatomy and physiology. I continued to read articles in renal journals and became excited to learn yet another mystery related to the kidney had been unraveled, particularly if the discovery was relevant to patient care. Indeed, the challenge of deciphering important interactions between the kidney and other organs was a major inducement for me and for others in electing to embark on a nephrology career. Second, as noted in various parts of this book, I cultivated a strong work ethic starting in grammar school. This gave me the strength and determination to put in the effort to excel in sports and in school. This sense of achievement raised my self-esteem and provided joy and fulfilment at a critical juncture in my social development. Similarly, I was convinced that the effort, financial investment, and length of time necessary to complete my medical school education would be eventually rewarded. Third, at the start of my career, I developed a strong drive to excel in my field, motivating me to establish several novel approaches that proved beneficial to children with diverse renal disorders. Witnessing the extent to which my medical interventions benefited my patients and receiving such gratitude from their families reinforced my sense of pride, fulfillment and enjoyment of my work. I also experienced a sense of accomplishment whenever one of my articles appeared in scientific journals and books or when other scientists confirmed my study results and conclusions. Fourth, because initially I was the only pediatric nephrologist in Western Pennsylvania and many children with life-threatening renal disorders depended on me, I had to be available to them continuously. As a result, I developed a strong bond with families that I believe is evident from their letters and patient anecdotes.

In summary, my motivation for hard work was driven by multiple factors, and my work became its own reward. I hasten to add, however, that neither my family nor friends (nor I, for that matter) ever considered me a workaholic, as I made time for my family as well as continued to participate and compete in various sports, encouraging both of our daughters to do so as well.

Although eligible by my age, prior to this time, I had not seriously contemplated full retirement. After forty-two years of practicing pediatric nephrology, setting the date of my retirement as February 28, 2017, imparted a sense of finality. As a formality, I was asked to submit a letter to my successor resigning my position (shown below). This was somewhat depressing and felt like the proverbial nail in the coffin.

12/13/2016

Dear Dr. Bates:

As we have recently discussed, I am resigning my employment from the Department of Pediatrics, the University of Pittsburgh, and the University of Pittsburgh Physicians effective 02/28/2017 (this will be my last day of work). I am also resigning my medical staff privileges at Children's Hospital of Pittsburgh as of the same date.

It has been a pleasure to work with you and my colleagues in the Division of Nephrology and the Department of Pediatrics. Thank you.

Sincerely,

Demetrius Ellis, M.D.

cc: Department Chair

Have I succeeded in life and professionally?

‌‌⸻

THERE IS A poem written by the famous poet, essayist, and philosopher Ralph Waldo Emerson that resonates with me because I strived to incorporate in my life most of the simple yet very meaningful measures listed. The teacher in me took the liberty of converting this into a quiz with an arbitrary score scale. I will not reveal my own score, but yes, I feel most successful and very content.

POEM ELEMENTS

	Weight	Grade 1-100
To laugh often and love much	15	
To win the respect of intelligent people and the affection of children	10	
To earn the approbation of honest citizens a nd endure the betrayal of false friends	5	
To appreciate beauty	10	
To find the best in others	15	
To give of one's self	15	

To leave the world a bit better,
whether by a healthy child, a garden patch,
or a redeemed social condition   10

To have played and laughed with
enthusiasm and sung with exultation   10

To know that even one life has breathed
easier because you have lived   10

This is to have succeeded

Albeit less elegant, I offer my own definition of success. In my view, success is meeting the challenge of one's existence: to use to the fullest all the physical and intellectual tools with which one is endowed by birth and subsequently modified by human experience, in order to accomplish one's dreams. Again, I conclude that I have succeeded.

Preview of my retirement

In retirement, I plan to continue participating in several sports that I have always enjoyed. Given my long and happy interaction with children of all ages during my pediatric career, finding a means for imparting my sports skills and experience through coaching of children is very appealing to me. Also, taking on a variety of projects has always motivated me in the past, and this book represents such a project. My hope is that this work may be of interest to our grandchildren in the same manner Irene's cookbook, *Irene's Recipes, With Love*, was dedicated to them and to our daughters. Hopefully, this and other projects will keep my mind occupied and sharp for the near future. In addition, as my daily biorhythms adjust, Irene and I hope to travel and spend more time together in places of interest. In addition, by convention, I must transition from being a taxpayer to becoming a Social Security recipient.

LETTERS FROM MY
COLLEAGUES AND FELLOWS

⁓

AS MY RETIREMENT date approached, I began to receive many amazing letters from former renal fellowship graduates and dialysis nurses. These were heartwarming and ego boosting, but beyond that, because I was so familiar with the individuals who sent them, I knew that they were not being frivolous with their compliments, and their genuine sincerity was evident in their words. A sampling of such emails and letters is included below:

Dr. Ellis

It seems unbelievable that your deep Greek laugh and authoritative voice will no longer be heard illuminating everyone about the intricate, ever fascinating detail of renal physiology. Has Children's Renal Division ever been without you? You have in fact been the constant for many years and it is your steadfast dedication that has allowed both the Renal Division and its associated disciplines to achieve such success. Your commitment to exemplary patient care and your enthusiasm for knowledge and teaching should be the standard by which clinicians practice medicine.

Personally, you will always have my gratitude for your mentorship. You not only created an exceptional fellowship for me, but you always offered your guidance and instruction. I am sure you played a large role in my being able to pass those challenging renal boards on my first try. I still remember how excited (and surprised) we all were to get those scores- and certainly remember that Irene baked a most delicious cake to celebrate!

I will always cherish my time with you as my teacher and my boss. You deserve a fabulous happy retirement.

With deep respect for all you have achieved, and great excitement for all to come.

Wishing you much happiness.

With love,

Susan (Susan Lombardozzi-Lane, M.D.)

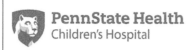

PennState Health
Children's Hospital

Michael Freeman
Penn State Hershey Children's Hospital
Division of Pediatric Nephrology and Hypertension
500 University Drive
Mail Code H085
Hershey, PA 17036
May 23, 2016

Demetrius Ellis, MD
Children's Hospital of Pittsburgh
Division of Pediatric Nephrology
One Children's Hospital Drive
4401 Penn Ave
Pittsburgh, PA 15224

Dear Dr. Ellis,

I have heard from MJ that you will be taking your well-deserved retirement this summer. I just wanted to take a moment to let you know that you will be sorely missed. My experience of learning under you as a resident is a large part of what led me to pursue my fellowship and I was delighted that I had the opportunity to continue as one of your mentee's as a fellow. Thank you again for all that you taught me, as well as countless other developing physicians over your many years.

Sincerely,
Your student

Michael Freeman

Dr. Ellis,

I heard from my dad that I am missing the celebration of your retirement this morning at CHP grand rounds. Congratulations! I know this, and every other celebration is well deserved.

Thanks,
Manu

———

"People will forget what you said, people will forget what you did, but people will never forget how you made them feel."
—Maya Angelou

Dear Irene and Demetri,

Thank so much for inviting us to Demetri's retirement celebration. We really enjoyed ourselves. Everything felt so comfortable and cozy and you looked so elegant.

We already know Demetri to be a warm, kind and loving friend with a generous spirit. But it was so affirming to hear his colleagues express their love and appreciation to him as they described him as an excellent and innovative doctor. They are so proud of him and clearly very proud of the two of you.

We wish you continued joy in your life together and with your family.

Warmly,

Dennis and Penny

Demetri,

We will miss you. You will never be forgotten. You have made an indelible imprint on the division, and we will maintain your legacy of high standards, innovative care, and dedication to patients and teaching. We will remain in touch, and I will send you updates. Thanks for all you have done in mentoring me and serving as an excellent role model.

Enjoy your retirement.

Mike

(Michael Moritz, M.D., Clinical Director, Division of Nephrology, CHP)

Dear Dr. Ellis,

It was an honor and pleasure to work for you. Enjoy your retirement and grandchildren. CHP has lost one of the best physicians.

Take care,

Nancy

(Nancy W. RN MSN CNS, former nephrology nurse and physician assistant)

Dear Dr. Ellis,

Congratulations on a wonderful nephrology career. You have given so much to so many.

I wanted to tell you that it has been an honor to have known you and worked with you and the children at CHP. I worked with you when CHP was in Oakland and Mary Hyrinia was in charge. Those were the days when we thought we could dialyze a neonate and then we did. It was successful, and the baby survived. Thank you for staying at the bedside with us dialysis nurses to encourage us, support us, and succeed.

I also worked with you at CHP when we moved to the New Campus in Lawrenceville. I was hesitant to come and work solely in pediatric nephrology, dialyzing only the children. But I must say that in my thirty-five years of being a dialysis nurse, being a pediatric dialysis nurse was extremely rewarding. I know what it means when it is said, "Let's take good care of the kids; they deserve no less than the best." And the best is what they got in you.

I have since returned to acute adult dialysis at Presby. Since I've worked there, I have met several now-adult patients who started dialysis as children. When I asked them, "Who was your doctor?" they said, "I started dialysis at Children's Hospital of Pittsburgh. My doctor was Dr. Ellis. He was great. I loved him. He would see me in clinic and I didn't want to cooperate at all. No blood work, no exam, no talking about what was wrong with me or what would make me better. Then Dr. Ellis would talk to me and he got me to do things I didn't really want to do. He was so nice to me even if I wasn't very nice to him back then." This might be the best compliment one could ever receive.

The children truly do love Dr. Ellis. How about the little boy who collected lanyards and you gave him the one you had around your neck? And the child who talked about a stuffed animal, and during the next clinic visit, you had a new one for her? There is so much more to treating a child's renal failure and that's respecting them as children.

So with your legacy of caring for the children and their parents, I salute you. And as for research and trying what has never been done before to make the life of a child better, I am happy to say I was your colleague. I was one of your dialysis nurses who was able to do the impossible because of you. Thank you.

Best wishes to you and again thank you for devoting your professional life to the children and their families.

Respectfully,
Susan C., RN
One of your Dialysis Nurses

Tue 4/4/2017
Dear Dr. Ellis,

It was so nice to see you and your lovely wife at your retirement gathering.

The stories that were told by your colleagues were heartwarming.

I wish that some of the senior nurses from the renal unit could have come to say goodbye.

Susan Carter really wanted to be there, but she had to work.

She was going to email you. Hopefully, you'll get it before your

UPMC email account closes.

I am so honored to have worked with you over the decades.

You know how much I love dialyzing the kids! (I miss them)

I still remember when you asked me if I would come to the new CHP to start up the dialysis unit.

You were my inspiration! It was an adventure! One that I will never forget.

I wish you well, Dr. Ellis. I know you are going to enjoy your retirement!

Elaine

Elaine L. BSN RN CNN
Living Donor Transplant Coordinator
Thomas E. Starzl Transplantation Institute

LETTERS FROM MY
PATIENTS AND FAMILIES

MANY OF MY present and former patients have succeeded in raising families and pursuing their own careers (sometimes medical). Indeed, this book is a celebration of human courage, mental fortitude, and resilience, which enables us to overcome adversity and strive to lead "normal" lives. I wish to acknowledge my patients and their families for contributing to my education and for helping me create the brand of pediatric nephrology that I practiced. In addition, having experienced helplessness on more than one occasion, I realize the value of maintaining a good balance between humility and victory in a medical sense. I also wish to thank all my patients, but especially the teenagers, for helping me remain in a perpetual state of adolescence and, thereby, never growing old.

Upon announcing my retirement, I received many uplifting letters from former patients and parents; a few are heart-wrenching. Some letters also included pictures, drawings and mementos. One package was send by a transplant recipient and included a hockey puck with a note on it indicating, "I dedicate this to Dr. Ellis who took care of me since I was born. I used it to score my very first hockey goal in high school". I treasured these letters the most because, as noted in the introduction to this book, I have chosen to judge my success as a physician largely based on how I have been perceived by my patients and their families. Thus, I elected to end my book by including a sampling of these letters. Although these letters were uniformly flattering and gave me great pleasure, the letters received from parents who experienced grief were perhaps the most telling and served as reminders of my human inadequacies.

Indeed, the words of my patients and the patient anecdotes I share with you herein, have a far deeper meaning. They not only validate all my efforts on their behalf but remind me what a privilege it is to be permitted to touch people's lives, one at a time. This transcends nephrology and is the calling of everyone involved in the medical profession. My wish is that the next generation of physicians will be rewarded as much by their own patients.

To my great surprise, among the letters I received was one from Noah and one from his mom (see p. 65, "*Noah's Princess*"). Noah was obviously apologetic about his "scribbling" and was clearly aware of his limited vocabulary and grammatical ineptitude. However, his sentiments were plainly evident by the number of hearts that he drew, and I found his few words to be extremely expressive and emotionally touching. Indeed "the heart is wiser than the intellect" (see, quotations, p. 203). Although he intended for his letter to be exclusively for my perusal, I am sure that Noah, his mom, and all my other patients would permit me to share these letters with the readers of this book:

Hello Allas,

Greetings your way. I hope you are doing fine! (not shown here is his drawing of a smiling face and numerous hearts with human features). I think I am fine but I don't have anything to do; no job, no work. I hardly want to come to my check-up because you are not there and it is not fun. You are my best doctor and you will always be. I like you very much. I wish I could see you again and again. Could you be in the next time when I have my apointment so I can see you again? Please, thank you.

Goodbye,

Your patient,

Noah

Dr. Lettuce (because that's what Gage called you when he was little!)

You are one amazing renal doctor! From the start of him being sick when he was 5 months old, and then had the nephrectomy at 7 months. Now he is 15 years old! Time has certainly flown by! We all appreciate everything that you have done for our family! You have gone above and beyond …You have explained things to me, so I was able to understand everything that was going on with Gage being so sick. We will never forget everything you have done for us! I have also had the pleasure of working with you as a staff nurse and won't forget asking me where the 24-hour urine collection was on a patient! You will certainly be missed so much by our family as many more families feel the same way. I hope that you enjoy what I have got for you (sports shirt for golf) and wish you the happiest retirement ever! You deserve it!

Gage and Tina (mom) speaking with one voice

Dr. Ellis-

We want to wish you well. May your retirement be filled with joy and a change in pace. We are honored to have been one of your patients. We will always be thankful for your encouraging Tanner to play soccer. He may never be the competitor you are, but he loves the game!

Best wishes,

Matt, Trace and Tanner K

Dr. Ellis-

Congratulations on your retirement. Children's Hospital will surely miss you. Being Nikki's doctor, you were amazing. You always gave us hope and we know that you care and wanted the best for Nicole; and 18 years past transplant she is doing well. Got married and through the gift of a surrogate has a beautiful 2-year-old little boy.

Enjoy your retirement. You truly deserve it.

You are one doctor we will never forget!

Bernie, MaryAnn and Nicole R

Dr. Ellis and Nephrology family,

When we first came to clinic, Erin was not only sick but a very insecure girl. Because of your dedication, love and support she realized she had become a "nephrology kid". To her that meant that she belonged, and you will take care of her. She was determined to do what you told her to do so that she would get better and she would not disappoint you. With your encouragement, she started seeing herself as you saw her- a great kid with a wonderful future. She once told me she felt she was given a second chance at life and will never take it for granted. When I look at Erin, I no longer see a little girl that hangs her head and never smiles but rather a young woman that holds her head up proudly and laughs.

The gift of money (graduation gift) you gave Erin was very generous but the gift you gave to Randy and I is priceless- you gave us back our daughter. We will never be able to repay you for all you have done but we hold you in our hearts and prayers always.

Elaine D

Dear Dr. Ellis,

When I first learned of your up coming retirement I felt sorry, for those children who will never know the doctor I did in my time of greatest need. I am over joyed to you, that you are retiring and you will have time for a whole new chapter in your life.

It has been over a decade since I first met you, and just a shade sooner since I last walked out of your office to head to adult clinic. I was one of your kids that graduated high school in 2004. I have the letter you wrote us to this day. I was not under your care long, just a short three years. I do remember never fearing my renal failure or my up coming transplant when you and I spoke about it. I was an emotional, frightened mess, when I first me you and I can never thank you enough to calming me and assuring me that it would be okay. That you would do what you could to help me. I don't remember everything from back then but I will never forget you.

I was in the hospital after my transplant for a long 21 days. It was absolute misery, I am sure that my mind has blocked out so much from those long weeks. I know that I was luckier than most children, and that in the great scheme of things and those few weeks where nothing. As a 16 year old that was an eternity. You where always brightening up my day with a Gardenia blossom, every morning that you came to check on me. It was rare that I was asleep during your visits, but when I was, I would wake and know you had been there with one on the bed next to my pillow. I am not sure if you knew how very much that meant to me, I knew that I always had someone on mine and my family's side during all of this. That you and your team where doing what you could. As you still do, and I am sure you always have done, for your kids.

It's been 14 years, this July, since my transplant. I can hardly believe that it's been so long. You will be pleased to know that I am doing great. My kidney is healthy as ever, adult clinic feels it will be there for the long haul. I am also happy to report that my hero, my donor Father, is doing great as well. We are closer than ever, and despite my age, I am still 'Daddy's Little Girl', truth be told I don't think he minds one bit.

When I was in high school I was in nursing at a vocational school, after I got sick, I couldn't bring myself to stay in the field. I was permitted to move to another part of that school, my hobby, art. I was always seen in clinic with my drawing pad and pencil. You sat me down when I decided to switch my major, you assured me that just because I was a transplant patient did not mean I could not still do what I wanted in life. Dr. Ellis, you told me that I could be anything, I still switched because Nursing was not my path. It seems, however, that art was not either. Shortly after dropping out of college with no real direction, my true passion was realized. With your words in my mind I started down another path all together, I attended a pet grooming academy, my mother and grandparents helped me start a business based around my grooming with a small retail attached. I worked for years along side of my Grandfather, he loved to help me with the 'big dogs' and we built the business together. He was proud of me and what we built together when he joined my grandmother in Heaven. I groomed for nearly a decade when I had complications with my hand and was retired out of grooming after surgery.

In those years that I was grooming, my Mom and I where also building that retail store. It quickly surpassed the grooming, so when I retired from my grooming career, I had a store to look after. Pet Parlor, is the name of my 'baby', it is not a large store but it means so much to me. I spend a lot of time researching natural and holistic foods, treats and health aide for all animals that I both share my life with and the ones my customers share theirs. I am now looking into training, dog training and cat behavior both, and I hope to one day do great things with my furry companions. I am starting with simple obedience and the basics in hopes to give our four legged companions hope from the start. I hope to one day work with homeless animals so they can find forever homes. My dream is to someday train dogs for search and rescue, cadaver retrieval and maybe even K-9 police. Nothing is paved in stone in life, and who's to say where training will take me.

For now I am going to continue building my store and hope that one day it will be a full 'pet store' where people can come and learn about their animal companions they are taking home. I don't want to be a store that is there for the sales, but for the animals, to teach children and adults proper care for their companions so they can live healthy and happily together. I share my home with a whole zoo of 'throw away' or 'misfit' animals that someone bought on impulse and forfeited because they did not realize or, more often, they where not taught the proper needs of the animals and they got to be too much. I have two Cavalier King Charles Spaniels, five domestic cats, one lion head rabbit, one bearded dragon, two millipedes, and aquariums. Don't worry Dr. Ellis, I am very careful with handling and cleaning. I live 'alone' from other people but I could not be happier with the family I do keep in my home. I feel that I was put here to help and work for the welfare for animals as you where for children.

Although much has changed as it will, I will always think fondly of my favorite doctor, Dr. Ellis. The kind man who supported me through my darkest and hardest trials of my youth, the same man I loved so much to make proud with doing everything he told me, and I hated so much to disappoint. You where a hero to a young girl that wasn't sure if she wanted to live or die. You are still to a woman who can always find you and your kindness in my heart. I knew you always believed in me even when I could not. I thank you deeply for that. Perhaps, one day we will meet again; I very much look forward to that day.

With all my love and respect,

P.S. The photos are with my 2 Cavaliers
Eve (white) is my girl
Xavier (black) is my boy

Dear Dr. Ellis,

It has been an honor to have you as Chris' doctor. You are the greatest. I even recommended you to a friend and they loved you also. You are always so kind and wonderful with Chris. He will always remember on the Nephcure Walk (organization promoting and funding causes important to kidney patients), when you took him and a couple other kids to the golf course. He enjoyed it. Chris was diagnosed with FSGS when he was 18 months, He had Rr. Moritz, Dr. Vats and then you. Between you and God, he is healed. The Cytoxan really helped him. He's been in remission since June 2012.

Thank you for everything.

Much happiness and health to you and your wife in retirement. Chris wrote:

Thank you so much Dr. Ellis for helping me through all of this. You really helped me, and I appreciate that.

Dear Dr. Ellis,

Thank you very much for your generous graduation gift. It was a delightful surprise to receive your letter. I recently learned that I'll be graduating at number six in my class, and I'm one of ten to receive the Presidential Academic Excellence Award. I am very excited to be attending the University of Pittsburgh next year. I hope to one day have as much of a positive impact on my patients as you've had on me.

Tara C.

Doc-

You have been there all my life and probably know more about me than I know myself. I hope you will continue to be there as I strive to become a pediatric nephrologist. My hope is to someday work under you as my guide. I'll miss you very much! And I'll make you proud.

John T.

Alex was twelve-years-old when she presented me an amazing poem that she had written and framed. It reflected her feelings after being diagnosed with systemic lupus erythematosus with kidney involvement. She responded well to therapy as described in p. 151 and eventually realized her childhood dream of becoming a literary author. Her freelance articles have appeared in *Cosmopolitan* and other publications. More than a decade after discharge from my service, I received the following letter from her parents along with an invitation to her wedding.

5/95

Dr. Ellis,

We are so very proud to send you this announcement (wedding invitation). You too, can share in our joy because of your major involvement. Carmine and I want to thank you for your knowledge, guidance, patience and compassion in the treatment for our daughter

Alexis. She can see some of her dreams come true because of your medical expertise. You are a very good doctor and person who we will be eternally grateful we met. We will <u>never</u> forget you or what you have done for our daughter, so she can lead a normal life.

Sincerely,

Carmine and Joyce D'A

August 3, 2005

Dear Dr. Ellis,

Thank you very much for the graduation money. It really comes handy because, even with college two weeks away, I have so much shopping to do! I would also like to thank you for being so in tune with me for all those years. I really appreciated having someone cheering for me when things got tough. I will keep in touch.

Sincerely yours,

Sarah D

11/29 2016

Dearest Dr. Ellis,

We don't know how to thank you enough for everything you have done for Brian! We wish you the best health, lots of family time, tennis, joy, love and – in your retirement. You know we will miss you very much and we hope that we can always keep in touch.

You have been more that Brian's doctor.

Brian, Karl Pat and ——

3/14/16

Dear Dr. Ellis,

It has been 21 years since my kidney transplant, and I am doing quite well to this day (only on 3 medications!). Thank you very much for your medical guidance, advice, and dedication from the beginning of my long medical journey!

You may recall in 2004-2008 I was doing my undergraduate degree at Carnegie Mellon University. After I graduated, I spent 5 years (2008-2013) at the University of Delaware and completed my Ph.D. in pure mathematics. In the following year, I spent a year working at the University of California, San Diego. I am currently working at the University of Maryland.

For the amount you have helped me, I am sure you have had an extremely positive impact on many of your other patients throughout the years. With new opportunities and experiences that lie ahead, I am wishing you the best in your retirement! Again, thank you very much for everything you have done for me!!

Sincerely Yours,

Dear Dr. Demetrius Ellis,

It gives me great joy to hear the news of your upcoming retirement! After 20+ years of unsurmountable dedication you have demonstrated to the profession I believe you deserve it sir.

After 20+ years of frequent biannual visitations, words cannot describe how much you have molded me into the man I have become today. You have inspired me to pursue my aspirations of pursuing medical school and helped fulfill my dream of becoming a doctor. I still remember you constantly expressing how blessed I am regarding my family, mild condition, and personal strength. You have always made sure I was keeping up with my medication regimen and demonstrated the importance of maintaining a healthy lifestyle.

As for me, unfortunately I underwent a total gastrectomy and lymphoma resection in 2013, however I am doing very well! I am finishing up podiatric medical school in Cleveland and moving to Pittsburgh to begin my 3 year residency training at Western Pennsylvania Hospital in July. I graduate May 20! I will be transferring my care from to Dr. Hariharan of UPMC. Even so, no one will be able to compare to the level of care I was provided by you.

It has truly been a pleasure getting to know you and having you as my pediatric nephrologist. I don't know where I would be to this day if it wasn't for your medical expertise, frequent life guidance, and words of encouragement. I hope to see you very soon. Congratulations on your retirement big guy and go enjoy yourself!

Warm regards, ____

REFLECTIONS OF "NEPHRON MAN"

3-14-15

Dear Dr. Ellis,
My family + I thank you
from the bottom of our hearts
for taking me into your care,
+ getting me on the right track
with my kidney disease. If it weren't
for you + your thoroughness, knowledge
+ passion for your patients, I
never would have been able
to live a normal life or have
a normal childhood. You saved
me from dialysis at a young
age + ever since then I have
been in good health. I am very
grateful to have had you
as my nephrologist for so
many years. You are most
definitely one of a kind
+ I will forever be thankful
for it. It's going to be
hard to match a new doctor
to you. I can only hope
to find another as wonderful
as you! We are sad you
are retiring, but you deserve
it! Thank you for everything!
I hope you find happiness in
your retirement + enjoy it!
(maybe play more tennis?)
GOD BLESS YOU! sincerely, ☺

Dear Dr. Ellis,

You will find us deep in your memory bank – Adam   and his family who only knew the DeSoto Street Children's. But we will always remember you as an integral part of our lives throughout Adam's childhood. We trusted you completely with his care. And seeing you always put us more at ease with what we faced.

We began the journey back in 1984 when Adam was 18 months old and you were with Dr. Ellis Abner. We stayed in a CHP ward with 4 patients per room - awful. The diagnosis: Focal Global Glomerulosclerosis – transplant in about 6 – 7 years. As predicted Adam had his first transplant (my kidney) in February, 1991. Adam enjoyed no school and endless popsicles from the floor kitchenette. FK506 was still in trial stage so we picked it up for free from Falk Clinic. To this day we call it FK and not Prograf. One of the enclosed photos is from that era at the annual Christmas party.

It became routine to head to CHP on many Wednesdays at 8:15 AM for bloodwork and waiting. During appointments you and Adam would talk about tennis and soccer, the sports you both played. You would comment that you always knew where to be on the soccer field but not on the tennis court. Then MJ would laugh and inform us that you, nevertheless, had won another tennis tournament.

It felt like smooth sailing until January, 1995. We came into clinic because I knew something was wrong – not just constipation as the ER had believed. Another diagnosis: We were told Adam was the first kidney transplant patient to have the Epstein-Barr Virus develop into Burkitt's Lymphoma. That was one rough year but the chemo didn't ruin his kidney. And while the oncologists took over his treatment we appreciated every time you looked in on him. Once you caught me checking drugs in a Physician's Desk Reference and advised me to "stop playing doctor." I'm sure I needed to hear that!

Seems like nine years is the span before Adam needs a new transplant. My sister donated #2 in the summer (2000) between his Junior and Senior years in high school. That one got him through college (Wittenberg University, 2005 BS in Chemistry) and graduate school (University of San Francisco, Chemistry.) During his first year (2009) working for Bayer Pharmaceuticals in Berkeley, CA he returned to UPMC for his third transplant donated by my dear friend. Haven't transplant procedures advanced through these years for both the donor and recipient!

The other photo shows Adam in 2013 with his kidney donors at his San Francisco wedding. We love Kassidy who understands all this chemistry talk. Adam now works for Simec Biomedical and says he can be as obnoxious as the rest of the Bay Area talking about their "start-ups." (But that's not Adam.) Both would move back here in an instant if there were pharmaceutical jobs in Pittsburgh.

Adam hasn't played tennis for years (hard on his knees) but still plays soccer (goalie) and ultimate frisbee. Until his office moves he commutes on his bike to the Ferry Building and across the bay – so California.

You will always be remembered fondly and with great respect. Thank you from the bottom of our hearts for your years of medical treatment and care. Enjoy your well-deserved retirement!

January 22, 2016

Dear Dr. Ellis

My sisters and I met you 23 years ago when they noticed Dawn's kidney issues, she was 11 years old. The next year they tested Danielle and Me and found we had the same kidney issues. Dawn was 13 when she had her transplant, which is still doing great. Danielle had her transplant when she was 14, which is still doing great. Then you get to me I've had three transplants to date, my first when I was when I was 15. Dr. Ellis you were there from the beginning until I was 21 year old. You helped us deal with the issues we had with a positive attitude and a smile on your face. You watched us all grow up.

Today Dawn and Danielle are 34 years old and both teachers, English and History respectively. Dawn graduated from college in December 2004 and received her Masters degree in 2012. Dawn is working full time at Jefferson Morgan Junior/Senior High School as a 7th/8th/9th grade English teacher. Danielle graduated from college in May 2006. Danielle is still looking for a full time position but she is subbing quite a bit. Today I am 31 years old. I graduated from college in May 2008 with a Sport Management degree. I got married on August 13th 2011 to a wonderful man Brandon Jacobs. My third transplant was on April 15th 2014. Now I am trying to recover from other health issues.

We would like to Thank You for your patience and presence in our crazy lives for so many years. Good Luck with your future! Happy Retirement!

Dear Dr. Ellis,

I want to thank you for being such an excellent, skilled doctor. You were my doctor from the time I was three months old until I was twenty years old. I had my kidney transplant when I was 21 months old and it is still working great. We celebrated the 20th anniversary of my kidney transplant in February. On May 7th, I graduated from Slippery Rock University with a Bachelor of Science in Business Administration. I graduated with highest honors, Summa Cum Laude. Ten people in the Business Administration program out of 158 graduated with highest honors. I want you to know this because I have worked really hard and want to succeed just like the role models in my life, such as you. I remember you were very caring and friendly and made me feel special every time I came to Children's Hospital. I hope you enjoy your retirement. I am very thankful you were my doctor over the years I went to Children's Hospital.

Dear Dr Ellis,

Congratulations! We understand that you have reached a milestone in your life – retirement! You are going to begin a chapter in your life that is well-deserved. Our lives have been enriched by knowing you and we wanted to bring you up to date with how knowing you has forever changed us.

Willie, now 38 years old, is married with a wonderful wife, Misty, a 14 year old step-son Jacob and a son, Trenten, who is 3 ½. We never thought Willie would live this long, let alone get married or have his own family. What a wonderful surprise Trenten was! The kidney Willie received in June of 1994 was truly a gift from God.

We remember that day as if it were yesterday. We had finished all the paperwork to have Willie put on the transplant list (somewhere around the 26th of May) but Holly did not give us a pager. She said that the odds of a kidney becoming available that quickly were slim to none and we had a vacation to North Carolina planned for mid-June. "Go on vacation and enjoy yourselves," she told us. So we did.

We arrived at Debbie's parents in Charlotte at 6 pm Sunday evening. At 6 am Monday morning, Debbie's mom woke us with the news that Pittsburgh was on the phone. Holly told us that there was a kidney for Willie. His reaction was to run out the door – after all, we were on vacation. What kid wants to immediately go back home – and for surgery? Holly told us we had 30 minutes to decide, but she said, and we quote "Dr Ellis says, 'come home, this is a gift'". We calmed Willie down and called Holly back and said "yes, we will be there."

From there, we needed a plane ride. Debbie's dad knew a US Air pilot who managed to get us 2 seats on an 8:30 am flight. Not only that, but the airport bumped all out-going flights so that our plane was first in line for take-off. Bill and Willie were in the air by 8:45 am. The other obstacle was how to get from the airport to Children's. Bill's niece had just been married the Saturday before and her new husband had to take his brother to the airport in Pittsburgh for a 10 am flight. "No problem," he said, "I'll wait for Bill & Willie and take them to the hospital." Problem solved. When Bill and Willie walked off their plane, Joe was waiting for them right across the concourse. They arrived at Children's by 11 am. Before the kidney.

You were right. This kidney was truly a gift. Willie had his transplant later that evening and had very few problems with his new kidney until just a few years ago. He had some rejection, which required some rigorous treatment, but Dr Shapiro managed to get it under control. He also began taking one of the newer anti-rejection meds in addition to his Prograf. His baseline creatinine is 2.5 – 2.8 which the doctors tell him is unheard of for a now 22 year old transplant.

We have had our bumps, but overall, Willie's life is good. You were right. This kidney was truly a gift. We can't say that often enough. When we first met you in 1978, we were young, scared parents with a sick child. Never in our wildest dreams did we think our lives would be like this. But your caring, your knowledge, your guidance, helped us raise a baby into adulthood. There have been times we were overwhelmed by the responsibility involved with having a sick child, but there was always someone at Children's to help us out. You and your staff were family to us at a time when the future was uncertain and we were scared.

We will miss you; but your retirement is well-deserved. May God richly bless you in all you do in the coming years.

Thank you!!!!!

Dear Dr. Ellis,

How are you? I hope this email finds you well.

My mom forwarded me the email of your reply to the one she had sent (I'm guessing with the photo attached) an I just wanted to take this opportunity to say thank you.

It goes without saying that none of this would be possible without your support, not only during my stint in London, but throughout the entirety of my life. My mom loves to tell the tale of how she came to meet you and how it really was destiny that things came to pass as they did. Well here we are years later, and I've graduated, and it really has to be said in a big way that I wouldn't be here without my family, you included Dr. Ellis because you've been ever mindful with me throughout the years , as much as a parent would be with their child as they grew and progressed through life. You've been with me during me highs and certainly been there to experience the lows too, and you have made me who I am now as much as these experiences have if not more.

For all of this I would like to just say thank you, I really could not have gotten this far without you, and certainly hope that you'll be with me for the following chapters of my life. Unfortunately, I haven't really had the chance to learn Hindi to find out and expression for the gratitude and support which I feel from you but I hope this will work too.

Thank you so much Dr. Ellis

Shabir

June 2016

Dear Dr. Ellis,

I really don't know where to start! I feel this letter deserves the personal touch as you give all your patients. Therefore, I am hand writing it instead of typing it. I feel you have given each and every one of your patients the feeling that they really matter. You take all the time needed to answer all questions that are asked, no matter how important they may seem.

I am able to write this letter to you all because "YOU" cared! Cody is a very healthy 15 year old. He will be going into the 10th grade for the 2016-2017 school year.

We met within a week of Cody's birth in May 2001. I was really scared as a first-time mother with a newborn that we weren't sure was going to make it. We traveled from ERIE to Pittsburgh. When Cody was brought to Pittsburgh and I met you, I knew he was in great hands. After the initial shock and immediate care was given, I felt a lot more relaxed.

You have saved my son's life with your expertise. Your knowledge allowed us to have ~~my~~ son thrive and grow into a teenager who is doing quite well. It really sticks in my head when you said he was a first to come off of peritoneal dialysis without needing a kidney transplant. To this day, I couldn't tell you how appreciative I've felt, knowing your care is why he's here and doing so well.

Because you have been so kind, caring, and taken

so much of your life to helping others, I wish you the best. I hope your retirement also allows you to enjoy many relaxing years of doing things you couldn't do as a full-time doctor. Please enjoy putting yourself, your wife, and family as sole priorities now. You deserve to do what makes you happy to the fullest.

We will all be sad to see you go, but you will always be in our thoughts and prayers. This includes everyone you have touched as being a doctor. You have been an exceptional doctor who has touched many lives, and I hope you feel your career has been beyond successful. You are one of our family members. You are a "One-of-a-Kind" individual!

"THANK YOU" from the bottom of our hearts. This just doesn't seem to be

enough for all you've done.
The World is a better place
with you as a person of
such wisdom & touching so
many lives. The   family
Wish you the best.

Many blessings to you,

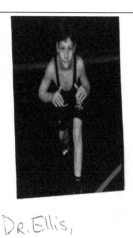

Dr. Ellis,

Just wanted to send a "Thank You" for all you have done during your career helping so many children and their families. Hope you can relax and enjoy your retirement.

Thanks again

It's nice to know that there are still people who take such pleasure in doing special things and making others feel good...

Thank You.
You're really someone special.

Thank you so much for doing so much to help Cody to be as healthy as he is today.